Cancer Screening Decisions

A PATIENT-CENTERED APPROACH

RONALD N. ADLER, MD, FAAFP

Associate Professor
Family Medicine and Community Health

University of Massachusetts Medical School
Worcester, MA

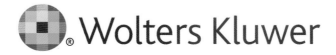. Wolters Kluwer

Start Here!

Cancer Screening Decisions

A PATIENT-CENTERED APPROACH

Deciding when cancer screenings are a good idea has never been more complicated. Patients are flooded with conflicting information about the value of screening tests and have no easy way to figure out if and when a screening test is the right choice for them. This book changes that.

CORE CONCEPTS

1 **Cancer screening can produce benefits, but also harms.**

2 <u>Patients</u> **should decide what cancer screenings they want based on:**

- *the best information available, presented in the clearest way possible*
- *their individual values and preferences*

This book is designed to:

- *provide the information needed, presented in ways that are Accurate, Balanced, and Clear*
- *illustrate the most important concepts*
- *communicate complex statistical likelihoods in visually engaging and illuminating ways*
- *serve as a tool to help clinicians guide patients through effective decision making — in ways that save time*

WHAT DOES SCREENING MEAN?

Screening means testing a person for a disease *while they do not have any signs or symptoms of that disease.*

If a woman has a lump in her breast, she should have a *diagnostic* mammogram to investigate the possibility of breast cancer. Though that is a mammogram, it is not considered screening. Similarly, a person with bleeding from the rectum should have a colonoscopy to investigate that; this also is not screening.

Throughout this book, only screening of *people without symptoms* is addressed.

THREE GENERAL TYPES OF CANCERS: TURTLES, BEARS, AND GRENADES

Many people erroneously think of cancer as a single disease with a predictable course: it begins small, gradually grows until it causes symptoms, and eventually — in the absence of treatment — will cause death. However, many cancers behave very differently. For example, cancer of the prostate is very different from cancer of the pancreas. Even within an organ, e.g., the breast, some breast cancers are aggressive and can be deadly, while many others are harmless: they would never cause death or any symptoms at all.

As a helpful analogy, throughout the book there are references to three general types of cancers:

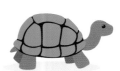

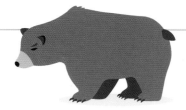

"TURTLES"

Cancers that are surprisingly common — *they move slowly and are non-threatening. They never cause death and don't even cause symptoms.*

Finding it early (or at all) is
NEVER HELPFUL

"BEARS"

Cancers that are potentially lethal, but often treatable, *especially when found early.*

Finding it early
MAY BE HELPFUL

"GRENADES"

Cancers that are very aggressive— they grow fast and are almost always deadly, even when found early.

Finding it early is
RARELY HELPFUL

CANCER SCREENING IS ABOUT TRADE-OFFS

We should think of cancer screening as being about *trade-offs,* because there are *benefits AND harms.*

This is what makes cancer screening decisions difficult — and is the reason that individual patients should decide for themselves. Reasonable people might feel that it is worth doing, while other — equally reasonable — people might not think it's worth it.

Most people — patients *and* clinicians — imagine cancer screening to produce more benefits and fewer harms than it really does. There are quite a few good reasons for this:

- *Our first cancer screening program, Pap testing for cervical cancer, has been highly successful, and we want to believe that other cancer screening programs will be equally successful.* In fact, Paps have been so successful due to the biology of cervical cancer: it grows very slowly and spends a long time in a pre-cancerous state when we can diagnose and treat it, preventing the cancer from ever developing. Unfortunately, the biology of other cancers is very different, so screening programs for other cancers have been less successful.

- *It is in our nature to assume cause and effect*, so when a patient has a cancer diagnosis after a screening test, and they survive, we assume that the screen was the reason: "early detection saves lives." Most of us know at least one cancer survivor, and these stories are very powerful. But it is not always the case that the screening test was the reason for the person's survival.

- *We are sometimes influenced by widespread media campaigns* that uncritically promote cancer screening — and cause us to be more accepting of associated harms.

Though medicine is very scientific, the best we can do in predicting what will happen in cancer screening involves *probabilities in a population* of patients. Because it can be difficult for many people to fully understand probabilities, we use pictograms throughout this book to *illustrate* probabilities.

UNDERSTANDING THE POSSIBILITIES

If you decide to be screened for cancer, the following chart outlines the possible outcomes. The outcomes after a true positive result are primarily determined by the <u>biology</u> of the diagnosed cancer, i.e., is it a Turtle, Bear, or Grenade?

Do false negatives ever happen?

Most negative results are true negatives, but *false negatives do sometimes occur.* In a false negative, the person has cancer, but the test misses it, and the reported result suggests that cancer is NOT there.

This can result in no harm or missed opportunities, depending on the type of cancer. It is another way in which screening tests may be inaccurate, but for simplicity, false negatives are ignored in this book.

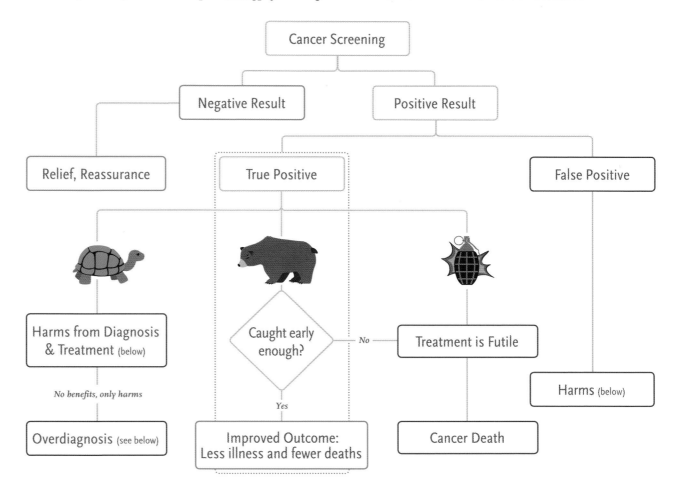

Cancer screening is helpful when:

1 A person without cancer has a negative (normal) screening test result

This is a small benefit that <u>many people</u> get to experience

2 A person with cancer has a positive (abnormal) test result, **_and_**

- the cancer they have is treatable, **_and_**
- they receive successful treatment, **_and_**
- the treatment is **_more successful_** than it would have been if the cancer was diagnosed later because of symptoms

This is a huge benefit that a <u>relatively small number of people</u> get to experience

This can only occur for bear-type cancers.

Cancer screening is harmful when:

1 A person experiences **_burdens of testing_**, such as inconvenience, discomfort, or large expenses

2 A person without cancer receives a **_false positive_** test result, in which her/his cancer screening test is abnormal, raising worries about cancer, resulting in:

- **_additional tests_**, which may cause more inconvenience, discomfort, and expense
- **_problems from more invasive tests_**, such as biopsies (minor surgery to remove a piece of the body for more precise testing)
- **_cancer anxiety_**, which can last for years after the false positive test result

3 A person experiences **_overdiagnosis and overtreatment_**: the diagnosis and treatment of a cancer that — if not for the screening test — would have never caused the patient any problem in their lifetime

Key: | Benefit | | Harm |

9

CANCER PROGRESSION *and How Overdiagnosis Can Happen*

To understand how overdiagnosis happens, one must appreciate the different ways in which cancers can progress. This is illustrated in the chart below, which shows that:

 Grenade-type cancers grow very fast and lead to early cancer death (dotted, red horizontal line).

 Bear-type cancers grow more slowly, and — through screening — can be diagnosed before they ever cause symptoms (dotted, yellow horizontal line). Sometimes this can lead to treatments that prevent death from cancer.

 Turtle-type cancers never advance far enough to cause symptoms or death — and they are available for a long time to be found by a screening test (if done).

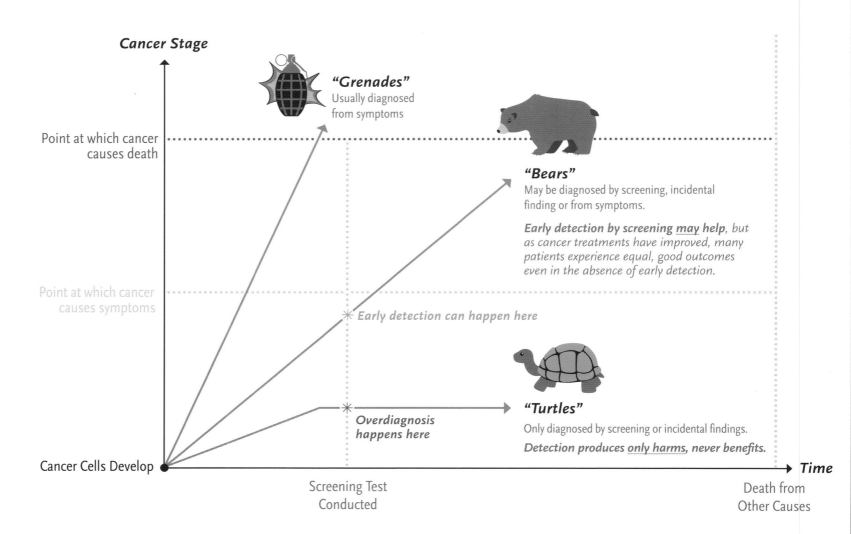

Overdiagnosis is the diagnosis of a disease that will never cause symptoms or death in a person's lifetime. It's the correct diagnosis, but irrelevant because treatment cannot possibly help the patient.

In cases of overdiagnosis, patients experience only harms — without benefits — from the diagnosis and treatment:

- **Physical:** injury, pain, or discomfort
- **Psychological:** anxiety
- **Economic:** cost, loss of future insurability or employability

The ideal screening program would find all of the bears and none of the turtles.

OVERDIAGNOSIS EXPLAINED

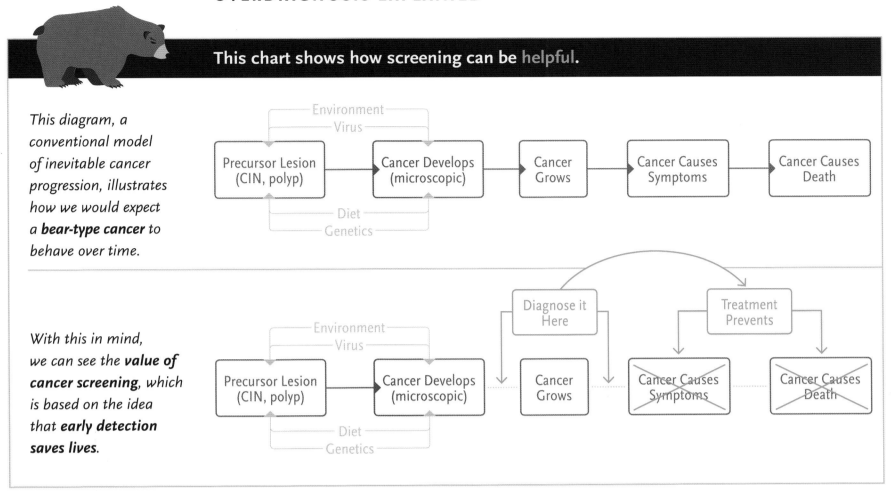

This chart shows how screening can be helpful.

*This diagram, a conventional model of inevitable cancer progression, illustrates how we would expect a **bear-type cancer** to behave over time.*

*With this in mind, we can see the **value of cancer screening**, which is based on the idea that **early detection saves lives**.*

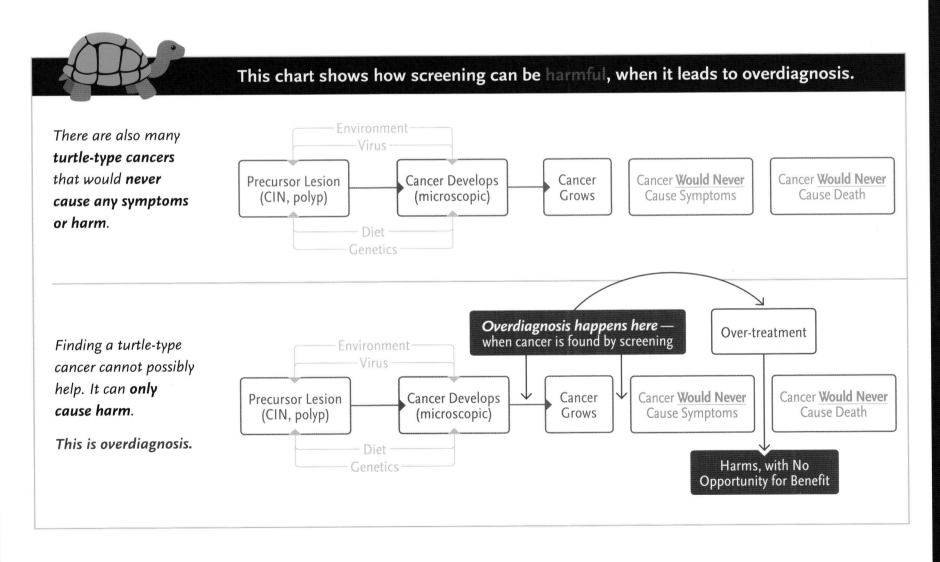

This chart shows how screening can be harmful, when it leads to overdiagnosis.

*There are also many **turtle-type cancers** that would **never cause any symptoms or harm**.*

*Finding a turtle-type cancer cannot possibly help. It can **only cause harm**.*

This is overdiagnosis.

WELCOME TO THE "GRAY ZONE"

Despite a growing push in the last thirty years for evidence-based medicine, it turns out that only a minority of health care interventions are precisely and unequivocally supported by evidence. Though evidence is used to inform nearly all health care decisions, it is relatively rare that the evidence is so compelling that it indicates a single best intervention to the exclusion of alternatives. Rather, there are inevitably *trade-offs*, in which one strategy provides some advantages while also including some disadvantages. We might think of these as "gray zones," in which there are multiple, valid, reasonable options. This is the case for many cancer screening options. Stool testing vs. colonoscopy for colorectal cancer screening is one example (*see pages 49-51*).

Because humans and health care are so complex, health care decisions are often made in these gray zones. In such situations, it is often the case that individual patient factors and preferences provide the most compelling reasons for one choice over another. Therefore, it is essential that clinicians encourage patients to participate in these very personal health care decisions. This process is known as shared decision making.

It takes collaboration to reach a decision

Clinicians share *reliable, evidence-based information* about cancer screening with their patients.

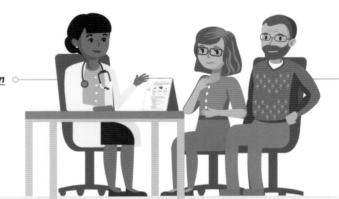

Patients explore and then apply their *feelings, values, and preferences* about the cancer screening choice.

SHARED DECISION MAKING

In shared decision making, a clinician shares information with a patient, who is prompted to consider his or her personal values and preferences. Armed with this information, the patient and clinician make a decision **together**. This is a core feature of patient-centered care; as such, it should be incorporated into routine care, including decisions about cancer screening. Unfortunately, shared decision making is underutilized, often due to barriers perceived by clinicians:

Clinician-Patient encounters should be approached as a dialog between two experts:

• **The health care professional** who has medical knowledge and expertise

and

• **The patient** who is an expert in his or herself and has a unique set of personal and cultural values

Myth	Reality
"Most of my patients just want me to tell them what to do"	Many patients would prefer to learn more about their choices
"I usually know what's best for my patients"	Evidence is often lacking, even for commonly recommended interventions, i.e. there are many gray zones
"The information needed to make decisions is too complicated to explain to most patients"	This book presents the information needed in easy-to-understand formats
"I don't have the time it takes to do this right"	This book includes decision aids that reduce the time required; other members of the health care team can be trained to use it with patients

12

SHARED DECISION MAKING: *Clinician Roles and Responsibilities*

① *Identify the need for a decision*

② *Invite the patient to participate*

③ *Frame the choice*

④ *Present the facts (Accurate, Balanced, Clear)* ○⸳⸳⸳

⑤ *Elicit patient values and preferences*

⑥ *Guide patient through the decision process, which may include deferring a decision*

> **Present the facts:**
>
> For the proposed test or treatment, explain the possible:
>
> • **Benefits:** the good things that can happen as a result of the test or treatment
>
> • **Harms:** the bad things that can happen as a result of the test or treatment
>
> • **Burdens:** the things the patient must do to get this test or treatment
>
> And also explain what is likely to happen to people who choose **not** to have the test or treatment.

This book will help the health care team accomplish these steps effectively and expeditiously, ultimately saving time. Each chapter has been designed to facilitate clear framing of choices on the first page with appropriate level evidence and information presented on the next page in a manner that is **A**ccurate, **B**alanced, and **C**lear. This enhances patient understanding and engagement, while standardizing the information presented to allow many different members of the health care team to have these conversations with patients.

SHARED DECISION MAKING: *Patient Roles and Responsibilities*

To choose the best option for you:

LEARN THE FACTS

• *Your risk* of the target disease, based on age, gender, and other factors

• *The potential benefits and harms* of testing

• *All the possible outcomes* related to being screened or choosing not to and the likelihood of each of these outcomes

• *Details of the test(s)*, including:

  • What happens to people who have the test, in groups of 1000, for example

  • Harms from the test (pain, etc.)

  • Accuracy of the test, including rates of false positive results

  • Likelihood of overdiagnosis

CONSIDER

• *Your feelings and preferences:*

  • How you feel about the disease and its treatment

  • How you feel about the test(s)

• *Your willingness to accept the risks* of testing in exchange for the possible benefits of reassurance or early detection

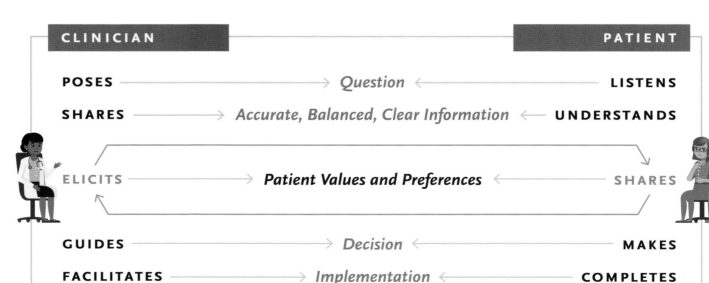

CLINICIAN		PATIENT
POSES ⟶	*Question* ⟵	**LISTENS**
SHARES ⟶	*Accurate, Balanced, Clear Information* ⟵	**UNDERSTANDS**
ELICITS ⟶	*Patient Values and Preferences* ⟵	**SHARES**
GUIDES ⟶	*Decision* ⟵	**MAKES**
FACILITATES ⟶	*Implementation* ⟵	**COMPLETES**

HOW TO USE THIS BOOK

The following pages contain a series of infographics that use the colors below to illustrate the potential harms and benefits of different types of cancer screening:

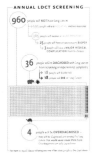

- **Gray:** No cancer
- **Green:** Cancer with good outcome
- **Black:** Cancer that results in death
- **Red:** Overdiagnosed Cancer (Cancer that would never cause harm if not diagnosed)
- **Yellow:** False Positive (= no cancer, but abnormal test result)

FOR CLINICIANS

This book was designed to stand between clinician and patient for simultaneous use. On the patient-facing side, there are large visuals and graphs. On the clinician-facing side, you will find a separate set of talking points to help you facilitate the conversation with your patient.

This book was designed to empower other members of the health care team to initiate complex conversations with patients about cancer screening. With some training and this book by their side, it is our hope that they feel confident to guide patients through the information, ask probing questions and provide accurate answers. If questions remain, the clinician can provide additional clarification.

We recommend displaying the books prominently in waiting rooms. Making copies available to patients who are waiting to be seen may "prime the pump" for constructive conversations.

BENEFITS OF DECISION AIDS

It has been shown[1] that people who use decision aids:

- Report higher levels of satisfaction
- Are less likely to remain undecided
- Feel more knowledgeable, informed, and clearer about their values
- Take a more active role in decision making
- Are more likely to make values-congruent choices
- Have a more accurate perception of their health risks

It is hoped that you, your staff, and your patients experience all these benefits.

ANNUAL CANCER INCIDENCE AND MORTALITY *(US, 2017)*

	Estimated New Cases			Estimated Deaths		
	FEMALE	**MALE**	**TOTAL**	**FEMALE**	**MALE**	**TOTAL**
LUNG	105,510	116,990	222,500	71,280	84,590	☑ 155,870
COLORECTAL	64,010	71,420	135,430	23,110	27,150	☑ 50,260
BREAST	252,710	2470	255,180	☑ 40,610	460	41,070
PROSTATE	—	161,360	161,360	—	26,730	☑ 26,730
CERVIX	12,820	—	12,820	4210	—	☑ 4210

☑ These numbers indicate deaths from cancers for which screening tests are widely available.

Source: American Cancer Society

1. Stacey D, Légaré F, Lewis K, Barry MJ, Bennett CL, Eden KB, Holmes-Rovner M, Llewellyn-Thomas H, Lyddiatt A, Thomson R, Trevena L. Decision aids for people facing health treatment or screening decisions. *Cochrane Database of Systematic Reviews* 2017, Issue 4. Art. No.: CD001431. DOI: 10.1002/14651858.CD001431.pub5

AN INTRODUCTION TO

Breast Cancer Screening

Clinician Talking Points & Discussion Guide

Below, please find suggested questions and talking points to help guide your conversation with your patient. If a bullet has a ★ next to it, we <u>highly recommend</u> including this in your discussion.

Introduction

Ask:

★ "Is this a good time for you to discuss breast cancer screening?"

• "Is there anyone else you would like to participate in the conversation, such as a family member?"

Set the Stage

Share:

• Breast cancer is the most common malignancy in women. Each year per 100,000 women in the US, there are about 125 new cases diagnosed and 21 women die[1].

• Rates have risen since 1980 due to the widespread adoption of screening mammography.

★ Breast cancer mortality has gone down, but **at least 2/3 of this reduction is due to improved treatments, rather than to early detection by screening**[2].

★ Many women with breast cancer experience the same (good) treatment outcome, whether it was detected by a screening mammogram or by noticing a lump. Thus, **early detection does not always confer an advantage**.

Review — This is what some of the "experts" say

Share:

★ Due to the epidemiology of breast cancer and predictable anatomic changes of the breast with advancing age, **mammography is a much better screening tool for older women than younger women**.

• The optimal screening interval between mammograms is not known.

Emphasize:

★ These recommendations are for **women who are NOT at high risk** of breast cancer.

  • Women at high risk include those who have preexisting breast cancer or a previously diagnosed high-risk breast lesion or an underlying genetic mutation (such as a BRCA1 or BRCA2 gene mutation or other familial breast cancer syndrome) or a history of chest radiation at a young age.

★ Having a screening mammogram should be a personal choice because it involves **trade-offs among the benefits and harms**. (See pages 18-19)

★ It is **up to you** to decide based on your values and preferences.

Breast Cancer Screening
for women who are not at high risk[1] of breast cancer

YOU HAVE A CHOICE.
Knowing the facts can help you choose the best option for you.

Learn about the good and bad points of screening mammograms.
Think about what's most important to you.

Do I <u>want</u> to have mammograms to check for breast cancer?

How do I <u>feel</u> when I have a mammogram?

If I choose mammograms:
• At what age should I <u>start</u>?
• <u>How often</u> should I have them?
• At what age should I <u>stop</u> having mammograms?

This is what some of the "experts" say, but you can see that there is disagreement among the "experts."

US Preventive Services Task Force[2]

Age 40 – 49: Consider having a mammogram every other year

Age 50 – 74: Have a mammogram every other year

Age 75 and older: Evidence is insufficient

Women get the best balance of benefit to harm when screening is done every 2 years.

American Cancer Society[3]

Age 40 – 44: Consider having a mammogram every year

Age 45 – 54: Have a mammogram every year

Age 55 and older: Have a mammogram every other year (every year if preferred)

Continue until life expectancy is less than 10 years

All women should be familiar with the known benefits, limitations, and potential harms linked to breast cancer screening.

ONLY <u>YOU</u> ARE AN "EXPERT" IN YOURSELF.
Breast cancer screening is a personal choice, so you should decide for yourself. To make an informed decision, weigh the **potential benefits** against the **potential harms**. ➜

Screening Mammography Effects in a Population, by Age[3]

Age	Br Ca Deaths Averted (per 10,000)	Number Needed to Screen (to prevent 1 Br Ca death)	False Positives, Annual Screening (per NNS)	False Positives, Biennial Screening (per NNS)	Biopsies, Annual Screening (per NNS)	Biopsies, Biennial Screening (per NNS)	Overdiagnosis Cases (per NNS)
40s	4	2439	1495 (61%)	1015 (42%)	171 (7%)	117 (5%)	10
50s	8	1299	796 (61%)	546 (42%)	122 (9%)	83 (6%)	8
60s	21	469	233 (50%)	159 (34%)	33 (7%)	22 (5%)	5

NNS: Number Needed to Screen to avert 1 breast cancer death.

1. U.S. Cancer Statistics Working Group. United States Cancer Statistics: 1999-2014 Incidence and Mortality Web-based Report. Atlanta: U.S. Department of Health and Human Services, Centers for Disease Control and Prevention and National Cancer Institute; 2017. Available at: www.cdc.gov/uscs

2. Welch HG, Prorok PC, O'Malley AJ, Kramer BS. Breast-Cancer Tumor Size, Overdiagnosis, and Mammography Screening Effectiveness. *N Engl J Med* 2016;375:1438-47.

3. Adapted from Nelson HD, Cantor A, Humphrey L, Fu R, Pappas M, Daeges M, Griffin J. Screening for Breast Cancer: A Systematic Review to Update the 2009 U.S. Preventive Services Task Force Recommendation. Evidence Synthesis No. 124. *AHRQ* Publication No. 14-05201-EF-1. Rockville, MD: Agency for Healthcare Research and Quality; 2016.

Breast Cancer Screening

for women who are not at high risk[1] of breast cancer

Learn about the good and bad points of screening mammograms.
Think about what's most important to you.

> Do I want to have mammograms to check for breast cancer?

> How do I feel when I have a mammogram?

> **If I choose mammograms:**
> - At what age should I start?
> - How often should I have them?
> - At what age should I stop having mammograms?

This is what some of the "experts" say, but you can see that there is disagreement among the "experts."

US Preventive Services Task Force[2]

Age 40 – 49: Consider having a mammogram every other year

Age 50 – 74: Have a mammogram every other year

Age 75 and older: Evidence is insufficient

Women get the best balance of benefit to harm when screening is done every 2 years.

American Cancer Society[3]

Age 40 – 44: Consider having a mammogram every year

Age 45 – 54: Have a mammogram every year

Age 55 and older: Have a mammogram every other year (every year if preferred)

Continue until life expectancy is less than 10 years

All women should be familiar with the known benefits, limitations, and potential harms linked to breast cancer screening.

1. Women at high risk include those who have preexisting breast cancer or a previously diagnosed high-risk breast lesion or an underlying genetic mutation (such as a BRCA1 or BRCA2 gene mutation or other familial breast cancer syndrome) or a history of chest radiation at a young age.
2. The USPSTF is an independent, volunteer panel of national experts in prevention and evidence-based medicine. For more information, visit www.uspreventiveservicestaskforce.org.
3. Oeffinger KC, Fontham ETH, Etzioni R, et al. Breast cancer screening for women at average risk 2015 guideline update from the American Cancer Society. JAMA 2015; 314(15):1599-1614

ONLY YOU ARE AN "EXPERT" IN YOURSELF.

Breast cancer screening is a personal choice, so you should decide for yourself.

To make an informed decision, weigh the **potential benefits** against the **potential harms**.

Review the Benefits of Mammography

Share:

⭐ There is **no all-cause mortality benefit** from screening mammograms.

⭐ The breast cancer mortality benefit from screening mammograms is **surprisingly small**[1]:

- Only 1 in 2439 for women in their 40s
- 1 in 1299 for women in their 50s, and
- 1 in 469 for women in their 60s.

• For many women, the **reassurance** of a negative mammogram is very important and helpful.

Review the HARMS of Mammography

Share:

⭐ Mammography is an imperfect tool; there are many false positive results, many of which lead to invasive biopsies.

⭐ The benefits of mammography — small as they are — come with some harms and risks.:

- ⭐ ALL women who choose screening will experience **the burdens of testing** (physical pain, anxiety, inconvenience, etc.).
- ⭐ About half of women who choose screening will experience **false positives** (leading to repeat mammograms or ultrasound +/- biopsies).
- ⭐ Very few women will experience **overdiagnosis of breast cancer** (leading to unnecessary painful, disruptive, disfiguring, costly treatments).

• Though we know overdiagnosis occurs in about 1 in 4 mammographically-detected breast cancers, we can never be sure which women were the overdiagnosed cases; they all get the same approach to treatment.

Emphasize:

⭐ Having a screening mammogram should be a personal choice because it involves trade-offs among these benefits and harms.

⭐ It is up to you to decide based on your values and preferences.

SURPRISING FACTS *about Mammography*

Though many women have avoided dying of breast cancer because a mammogram found breast cancer early, when we look at a large group of women, we see that

SCREENING MAMMOGRAMS:

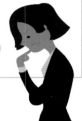

1 ARE *less helpful* THAN WE THOUGHT

2 CAN *lead to harms* FOR MANY WOMEN

HARMS
(some of which are minor and others are very bad)

1 BURDENS OF TESTING
- INCONVENIENCE
- DISCOMFORT/PAIN
- ANXIETY
- COST

2 FALSE POSITIVES
When abnormalities are seen and more testing is recommended, but **THERE IS NO CANCER**. The extra testing could be:
↳ a **repeat mammogram** with additional x-ray views or an ultrasound
↳ a **biopsy**, which is a surgical procedure in which a small part of the breast is removed.

3 OVERDIAGNOSED CANCER
Diagnosis and treatment of a cancer that **WOULD NEVER HAVE CAUSED SYMPTOMS, HARM, OR DEATH**; if not for the mammogram, the woman never would have found out about it — and never would have had a problem from it.

LEARN MORE TO MAKE AN INFORMED DECISION.
On the next page, learn more about the different general "types" of breast cancer. ➔

---

*Sometimes people wonder about the risk of the radiation from mammograms (which involve x-rays) **causing** breast cancer. There is a risk of this, but it is quite small, no more than 1 per 1000 women having annual mammograms from age 40 to 80.*

This risk may be reduced fivefold for women who choose biennial mammograms starting at age 50 compared to women having annual mammograms starting at age 40[2].

---

1. Adapted from Nelson HD, Cantor A, Humphrey L, Fu R, Pappas M, Daeges M, Griffin J. Screening for Breast Cancer: A Systematic Review to Update the 2009 U.S. Preventive Services Task Force Recommendation. Evidence Synthesis No. 124. *AHRQ* Publication No. 14-05201-EF-1. Rockville, MD: Agency for Healthcare Research and Quality; 2016.

2. Miglioretti DL, Lange J, van den Broek JJ, et al.: Radiation-Induced Breast Cancer Incidence and Mortality From Digital Mammography Screening: A Modeling Study. *Ann Intern Med* 164 (4): 205-14, 2016

SURPRISING FACTS *about Mammography*

Though many women have avoided dying of breast cancer because a mammogram found breast cancer early, when we look at a large group of women, we see that

SCREENING MAMMOGRAMS:

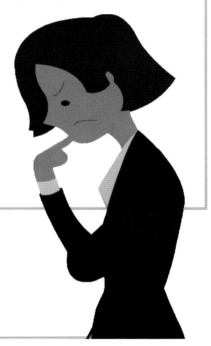

1 ARE *less helpful* THAN WE THOUGHT

2 CAN *lead to harms* FOR MANY WOMEN

HARMS
(some of which are minor and others are very bad)

1 BURDENS OF TESTING
- INCONVENIENCE
- DISCOMFORT/PAIN
- ANXIETY
- COST

2 FALSE POSITIVES
When abnormalities are seen and more testing is recommended, but **THERE IS NO CANCER.** The extra testing could be:
↳ a **repeat mammogram** with additional x-ray views or an ultrasound
↳ **a biopsy**, which is a surgical procedure in which a small part of the breast is removed.

3 OVERDIAGNOSED CANCER
Diagnosis and treatment of a cancer that **WOULD NEVER HAVE CAUSED SYMPTOMS, HARM, OR DEATH**; if not for the mammogram, the woman never would have found out about it — and never would have had a problem from it.

LEARN MORE TO MAKE AN INFORMED DECISION.

On the next page, learn more about the different general "types" of breast cancer.

Set the Stage

Emphasize:

★ **Breast cancer is not 1 disease:** some types are very aggressive and deadly, while others are so mild, they would NEVER cause ANY problem.

• To illustrate the point, we can think of the different cancers as Turtles, Bears, and Grenades. See pages 8-11 for more details on this.

Review "TURTLES"

Share:

★ Breast cancer is a heterogeneous disease: some breast cancers are very aggressive, while others are harmless: they would **never** cause symptoms or problems in a woman's lifetime. We can think of these as turtle-type cancers.

Dive into the concept of Overdiagnosis. See pages 10-11.

★ **Diagnosing and treating indolent (turtle) cancers only causes harm** – without any opportunity for benefit. This is overdiagnosis and overtreatment.

★ Overdiagnosis is surprisingly common in screen-detected breast cancers, accounting for about 25% with some estimates as high as 54%.

Review "BEARS"

Share:

• When people think of cancer, they are usually assuming bear-type behavior: a cancer that is biologically programmed to advance in a way that it will cause symptoms and eventually death if not successfully treated.

• These are the breast cancers for which mammograms are most important and useful, because early detection can substantially improve outcomes in some cases.

Review "GRENADES"

Share:

• These are the worst types of cancer.

• There is usually very little that can be done for women with such aggressive breast cancers — regardless of when it is diagnosed.

• Our best hope for these is the development of better treatments.

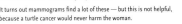

TYPES OF BREAST CANCER

"TURTLES"

Breast cancer that is surprisingly common — it moves slowly and is non-threatening. It never causes death and doesn't even cause symptoms.

It turns out mammograms find a lot of these — but this is not helpful, because a turtle cancer would never harm the woman.

THERE IS NO BENEFIT IN FINDING OR TREATING THESE CANCERS, AND THERE CAN ONLY BE HARMS: the woman gets cancer treatment, which typically involves a combination of surgery, radiation, chemotherapy, and hormones. We call this overdiagnosis and overtreatment.

"BEARS"

Breast cancer that is potentially lethal, but often treatable, especially when found early.

When it's small, we could kill it (i.e., treat it successfully), but when it grows too big and spreads, it's harder to treat and may kill the patient.

MAMMOGRAMS CAN BE VERY HELPFUL for these types of cancer, because they help us find them when they are small: Early detection may help avoid some breast cancer deaths.

One of the reasons mammograms are less helpful than we thought is because breast cancer treatments have improved so much that even when many bear cancers are found late (for example because a lump is felt), treatment may still be successful.

"GRENADES"

Breast cancer that is very aggressive — it grows fast and is almost always deadly, even when found early.

MAMMOGRAMS ARE NOT HELPFUL for this type of breast cancer. In fact, these are sometimes known as "interval cancers," because they appear in the interval between mammograms, that is, after a negative (normal) mammogram.

HOW WILL YOU DECIDE?
On the following pages, learn more about your chances of having a false positive, being overdiagnosed for breast cancer, and dying from breast cancer. ➔

21

Quick Summary

 Turtles: *Never Harmful*

 Bears: *Potentially Lethal*

 Grenades: *Always Lethal*

The type of breast cancer a woman has is usually the most important determinant of her prognosis.

The ideal screening program would find ALL of the Bears and NONE of the Turtles.

When a breast cancer is first diagnosed, it is often difficult for doctors to determine whether it is most likely to behave as a Turtle, Bear, or Grenade.

New research is seeking to identify biological markers that can help address this question *— For a deeper understanding of this, see Lannin DR, Wang S. Are small breast cancers good because they are small or small because they are good? N Engl J Med 2017;376:2286-91.*

Women will have better outcomes when we can tailor treatment to provide more intensive treatment to those with aggressive cancers and less intensive approaches to women with cancers more likely to be indolent.

TYPES OF BREAST CANCER

"TURTLES"

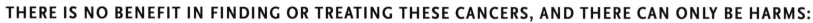

Breast cancer that is surprisingly common — it moves slowly and is non-threatening. It never causes death and doesn't even cause symptoms.

It turns out mammograms find a lot of these — but this is not helpful, because a turtle cancer would never harm the woman.

THERE IS NO BENEFIT IN FINDING OR TREATING THESE CANCERS, AND THERE CAN ONLY BE HARMS: the woman gets cancer treatment, which typically involves a combination of surgery, radiation, chemotherapy, and hormones. We call this overdiagnosis and overtreatment.

"BEARS"

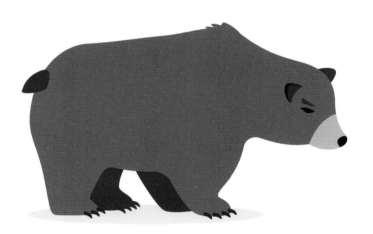

Breast cancer that is potentially lethal, but often treatable, especially when found early.

When it's small, we could kill it (i.e., treat it successfully), but when it grows too big and spreads, it's harder to treat and may kill the patient.

MAMMOGRAMS CAN BE VERY HELPFUL for these types of cancer, because they help us find them when they are small: Early detection may help avoid some breast cancer deaths.

One of the reasons mammograms are less helpful than we thought is because breast cancer treatments have improved so much that even when many bear cancers are found late (for example because a lump is felt), treatment may still be successful.

"GRENADES"

Breast cancer that is very aggressive — it grows fast and is almost always deadly, even when found early.

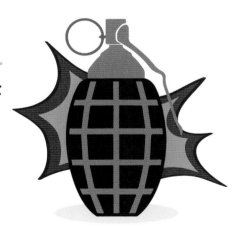

MAMMOGRAMS ARE NOT HELPFUL for this type of breast cancer. In fact, these are sometimes known as "interval cancers," because they appear in the interval between mammograms, that is, after a negative (normal) mammogram.

HOW WILL YOU DECIDE?

On the following pages, learn more about your chances of having a false positive, being overdiagnosed for breast cancer, and dying from breast cancer. ➡

Breast Cancer Screening

FOR WOMEN IN THEIR 40s

Clinician Talking Points & Discussion Guide

Below, please find suggested questions and talking points to help guide your conversation with your patient.
If a bullet has a ★ next to it, we <u>highly recommend</u> including this in your discussion.

Introduction

Ask:

★ "Is this a good time for you to discuss breast cancer screening?"

• "Is there anyone else you would like to participate in the conversation, such as a family member?"

Set the Stage

Share:

★ Each chart shows 10,000 women and what happens to them over 10 years based on whether they choose regular mammograms or not.

★ *Explain the meaning of the different color dots:*
  • Green: cancer with good outcome
  • Black: Cancer that causes death

• Though not shown in the charts, in these groups of 10,000 women, there are other cases of breast cancer — some diagnosed and some not — that do not cause death.

Review ANNUAL SCREENING vs. NO SCREENING

Share:

★ There is **no all-cause mortality benefit** from screening mammograms.

• The <u>breast cancer mortality benefit</u> from screening mammograms is **surprisingly small:**
  • Only 1 in 2439 for women in their 40s
  • This is approximated in the chart as 4 in 10,000 women who avoid dying of breast cancer due to having regular mammograms.

• This benefit —small as it is — comes with harms and risk:
  • The burdens of testing (physical pain, anxiety, inconvenience)
  • The risk of false positives (leading to repeat mammograms or ultrasound +/- biopsies)
  • The risk of overdiagnosis (unnecessary painful, disruptive, disfiguring, costly treatments)

Emphasize:

★ Each dot represents 1 woman, and each chart shows what happens to 10,000 women.

★ **You have an equal chance of being any one of the 10,000 dots.** Your choice is about whether you want to be in the group on the left or the group on the right.

• The left side shows a group of 10,000 women who choose regular mammograms.
  • In this group, there will be 30 women who will be diagnosed with breast cancer in their 40s and eventually die of breast cancer.
  • Because of mammograms, 4 out of 10,000 women avoid this.

• On the right side we see 10,000 women who choose to NOT have mammograms.
  • 34 of these women will be diagnosed with breast cancer in their 40s and eventually die of breast cancer.

★ Having a screening mammogram should be a personal choice because it involves <u>trade-offs among these benefits and harms</u>.

• It is <u>up to **you**</u> to decide based on your values and preferences.

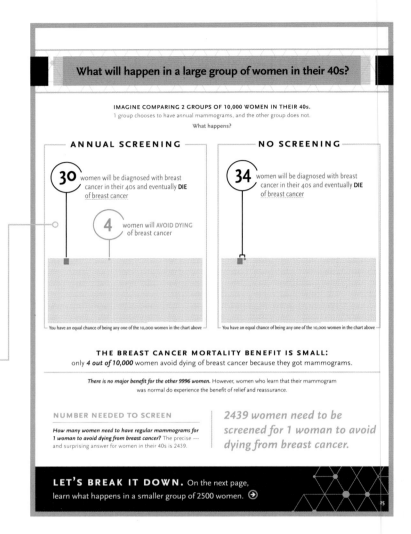

In 2016, the USPSTF stated that women ages 40 to 49 should ***"make their own decision whether and when to get a mammogram, in consultation with their doctors.*** This decision should be based on their health history, preferences, and how they value the potential benefits and harms of screening[1]."

Data for chart adapted from Nelson HD, Cantor A, Humphrey L, Fu R, Pappas M, Daeges M, Griffin J. Screening for Breast Cancer: A Systematic Review to Update the 2009 U.S. Preventive Services Task Force Recommendation. *Evidence Synthesis No. 124. AHRQ* Publication No. 14-05201-EF-1. Rockville, MD: Agency for Healthcare Research and Quality; 2016.

1. Albert L. Siu, MD, MSPH; on behalf of the U.S. Preventive Services Task Force. Screening for Breast Cancer: U.S. Preventive Services Task Force Recommendation Statement. *Ann Intern Med.* 2016;164:279-296. doi:10.7326/M15-2886

What will happen in a large group of women in their 40s?

IMAGINE COMPARING 2 GROUPS OF 10,000 WOMEN IN THEIR 40s.
1 group chooses to have annual mammograms, and the other group does not.

What happens?

ANNUAL SCREENING

30 women will be diagnosed with breast cancer in their 40s and eventually **DIE** of breast cancer

4 women will **AVOID DYING** of breast cancer

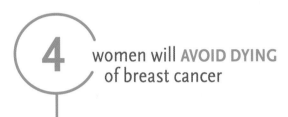

You have an equal chance of being any one of the 10,000 women in the chart above

NO SCREENING

34 women will be diagnosed with breast cancer in their 40s and eventually **DIE** of breast cancer

You have an equal chance of being any one of the 10,000 women in the chart above

THE BREAST CANCER MORTALITY BENEFIT IS SMALL:
only *4 out of 10,000* women avoid dying of breast cancer because they got mammograms.

There is no major benefit for the other 9996 women. However, women who learn that their mammogram was normal do experience the benefit of relief and reassurance.

NUMBER NEEDED TO SCREEN

How many women need to have regular mammograms for 1 woman to avoid dying from breast cancer? The precise and surprising answer for women in their 40s is 2439.

2439 women need to be screened for 1 woman to avoid dying from breast cancer.

LET'S BREAK IT DOWN. On the next page, learn what happens in a smaller group of 2500 women.

Set the Stage

Share:

★ These charts show a little more of what happens to a group of women who choose regular mammograms. This time, we are looking at **2 groups of 2500 women.**

• The group on the left has chosen to <u>have</u> regular screening mammograms.

• The group on the right has chosen to <u>not</u> have regular screening mammograms.

★ Each dot represents 1 woman.

★ You have an **equal chance** of being any one of the women represented by the 2500 dots.

★ In **each** group of 2500 women, 2463 women will not have or get breast cancer, and 37 (28 + 9) will have or get breast cancer.

★ **9 of the 37 breast cancers are turtle-type cancers:** they will not be diagnosed in the No Screening group — and they will never cause any symptoms or harm for those 9 women.

Review the ANNUAL SCREENING Section

• Among the 2463 women without breast cancer, the 930 gray dots (38%) represent women who will have consistently **negative mammograms.**

★ The 1533 yellow dots (62%) represent women who will have false positive mammograms.

★ **Explain the false positives**: things that are seen on the mammogram that raise a concern of a problem, but after further testing we learn that it was really nothing.

   ★ All 1533 of these women get extra testing; for most of them it is additional imaging tests, such as focused mammogram views or ultrasounds, but:

      ★ **175 will have a biopsy** (a surgical procedure to remove a sample of the breast to examine it under a microscope).

★ Among the 28 women with bad cancers (bears and grenades), the 20 green dots represent women who will **survive** and the **8 black dots** represent women who will **die** of breast cancer. <u>This is the prime benefit of screening, because 1 fewer woman dies</u> compared to the No Screening group.

★ The **9 red dots represent cases of overdiagnosed breast cancers:** <u>turtle-type cancers that were found only because of the screening.</u>

   • Because these never would have caused symptoms or harm, there is <u>no possible benefit from diagnosing or treating them.</u> Cancer treatments always cause harms. These women will die from something other than breast cancer.

★ **REMEMBER:** At the time of choosing screening, you have an <u>equal chance of being any of the women represented by these 2500 dots.</u>

Review the NO SCREENING Section

• The 2463 gray dots represent the women who do not have or get breast cancer. They have no testing and no problems.

• There are 28 women who will have or get a bad breast cancer (bear- and grenade-type). After developing symptoms, such as a lump, they will get diagnosed with and treated for breast cancer.

   • The 19 green dots represent women who will **survive**

   • The **9 black dots** represent women who will **die** of breast cancer, **1 more than in the screened group**

★ The 9 green dots in their own section represent turtle-type cancers, which will never cause any symptoms or harm. Because there is no screening in this group, they will never be found, so <u>these 9 women will not be harmed by unnecessary treatments.</u>

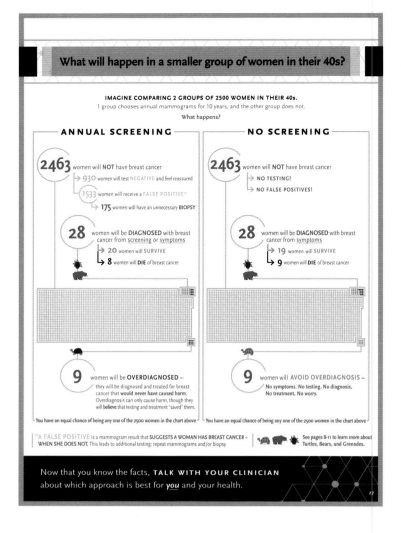

Comments on the Data

• For clarity of presentation, some numbers have been rounded.

• If screening is done <u>every other year,</u> there would be <u>fewer</u> false positives (1040) and unnecessary biopsies (120). See page 29.

• Rates of overdiagnosis have been reported over a wide range (0 – 54%), and the precise rate is not known. Evidence from the best designed studies suggest that at least 20% of screen-detected breast cancers represent overdiagnosis.[1,2,3] In this book, a rate of 25% has been assumed.

Data for chart adapted from:

Nelson HD, Cantor A, Humphrey L, Fu R, Pappas M, Daeges M, Griffin J. Screening for Breast Cancer: A Systematic Review to Update the 2009 U.S. Preventive Services Task Force Recommendation. Evidence Synthesis No. 124. *AHRQ* Publication No. 14-05201-EF-1. Rockville, MD: Agency for Healthcare Research and Quality; 2016.

Howlader N, Noone AM, Krapcho M, Miller D, Bishop K, Kosary CL, Yu M, Ruhl J, Tatalovich Z, Mariotto A, Lewis DR, Chen HS, Feuer EJ, Cronin KA (eds). *SEER Cancer Statistics Review,* 1975-2014, National Cancer Institute. Bethesda, MD, https://seer.cancer.gov/csr/1975_2014/, based on November 2016 SEER data submission, posted to the SEER web site, April 2017.

Hubbard RA, Kerlikowske K, Flowers CI, et al. Cumulative probability of false-positive recall or biopsy recommendation after 10 years of screening mammography: a cohort study. *Ann Intern Med.* 2011;155(8): 481-92. PMID: 22007042.

1. Bleyer A, Welch HG: Effect of three decades of screening mammography on breast-cancer incidence. *N Engl J Med* 367 (21): 1998-2005, 2012.

2. Kalager M, Zelen M, Langmark F, et al.: Effect of screening mammography on breast-cancer mortality in Norway. *N Engl J Med* 363 (13): 1203-10, 2010.

3. Jørgensen KJ, Gøtzsche PC: Overdiagnosis in publicly organised mammography screening programmes: systematic review of incidence trends. *BMJ* 339: b2587, 2009.

IMAGINE COMPARING 2 GROUPS OF 2500 WOMEN IN THEIR 40s.

1 group chooses annual mammograms for 10 years, and the other group does not.

What happens?

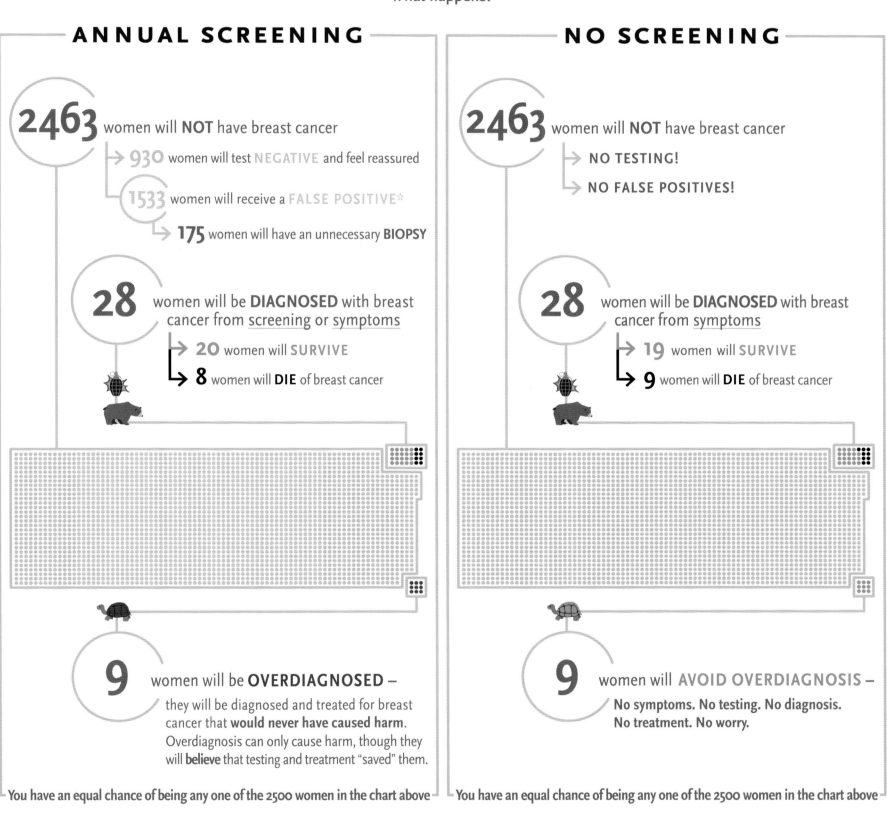

ANNUAL SCREENING

2463 women will **NOT** have breast cancer

→ 930 women will test NEGATIVE and feel reassured

→ 1533 women will receive a FALSE POSITIVE*

→ 175 women will have an unnecessary BIOPSY

28 women will be **DIAGNOSED** with breast cancer from screening or symptoms

→ 20 women will SURVIVE

→ 8 women will DIE of breast cancer

9 women will be **OVERDIAGNOSED** –

they will be diagnosed and treated for breast cancer that **would never have caused harm**. Overdiagnosis can only cause harm, though they will **believe** that testing and treatment "saved" them.

You have an equal chance of being any one of the 2500 women in the chart above

NO SCREENING

2463 women will **NOT** have breast cancer

→ NO TESTING!

→ NO FALSE POSITIVES!

28 women will be **DIAGNOSED** with breast cancer from symptoms

→ 19 women will SURVIVE

→ 9 women will DIE of breast cancer

9 women will AVOID OVERDIAGNOSIS –

No symptoms. No testing. No diagnosis. No treatment. No worry.

You have an equal chance of being any one of the 2500 women in the chart above

*A FALSE POSITIVE is a mammogram result that **SUGGESTS A WOMAN HAS BREAST CANCER – WHEN SHE DOES NOT.** This leads to additional testing: repeat mammograms and/or biopsy.

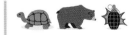 See pages 8-11 to learn more about Turtles, Bears, and Grenades.

Now that you know the facts, **TALK WITH YOUR CLINICIAN** about which approach is best for *you* and your health.

Set the Stage

Share:

- This page helps you compare 3 different strategies or approaches. The numbers show what happens to 3 groups of 2500 women in their 40s.

★ "As we look at these, consider which one feels most appropriate FOR YOU. **I am happy to support whatever choice you make.**"

Review the REGULAR SCREENING Section

Share:

- The first 2 rows show the outcomes for women who choose screening mammograms.
  - In the first row, women are getting a mammogram <u>every year</u>.
  - In the second row, women are getting a mammogram <u>every other year</u>.

★ The main differences are <u>fewer false positives and biopsies</u> in the group that has mammograms every other year.

Review the NO SCREENING Section

Share:

- In the last row, we see what happens to 2500 women who choose to not have screening mammograms.

★ You can see that they avoid false positives, unnecessary biopsies, and overdiagnosed cases of breast cancer, but <u>1 more woman dies of breast cancer in this group</u>.

- This is just 1 extra breast cancer death **per 2500 women**, and

- There is **no difference in all-cause mortality**.

Emphasize:

★ When considering whether you want a screening mammogram, there is no one "right" answer.

★ **The best decision is the one that feels most comfortable to <u>you</u>.**

Review the HOW SHOULD YOU DECIDE? Section

Share:

★ You might find it helpful to consider some of these questions.

Ask:

- Do you have any questions for me?
- Do you feel ready to make a decision?

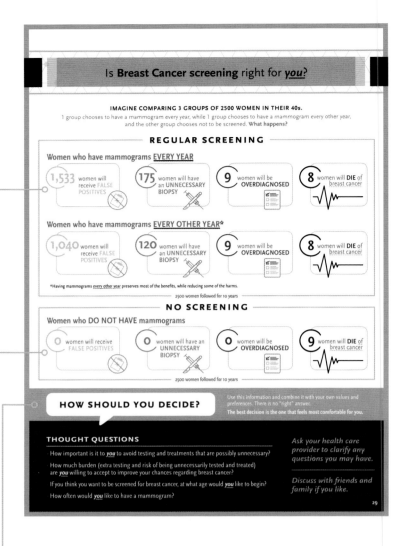

Did you know? False positive rates are > 20% higher in obese women[1].

1. Elmore JG, Carney PA, Abraham LA, et al.: The association between obesity and screening mammography accuracy. Arch Intern Med 164 (10): 1140-7, 2004

Is **Breast Cancer screening** right for *you*?

IMAGINE COMPARING 3 GROUPS OF 2500 WOMEN IN THEIR 40s.

1 group chooses to have a mammogram every year, while 1 group chooses to have a mammogram every other year, and the other group chooses not to be screened. **What happens?**

REGULAR SCREENING

Women who have mammograms <u>EVERY YEAR</u>

1,533 women will receive FALSE POSITIVES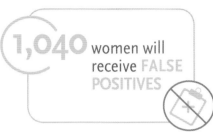

175 women will have an UNNECESSARY BIOPSY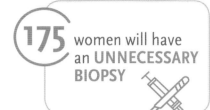

9 women will be OVERDIAGNOSED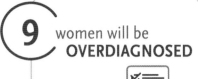

8 women will **DIE** of breast cancer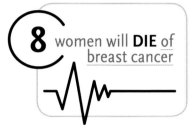

Women who have mammograms <u>EVERY OTHER YEAR</u>✳

1,040 women will receive FALSE POSITIVES

120 women will have an UNNECESSARY BIOPSY

9 women will be OVERDIAGNOSED

8 women will **DIE** of breast cancer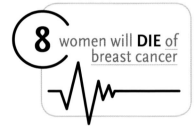

✳Having mammograms <u>every other year</u> preserves most of the benefits, while reducing some of the harms.

— 2500 women followed for 10 years —

NO SCREENING

Women who DO NOT HAVE mammograms

0 women will receive FALSE POSITIVES

0 women will have an UNNECESSARY BIOPSY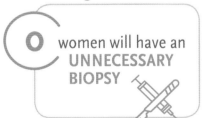

0 women will be OVERDIAGNOSED

9 women will **DIE** of breast cancer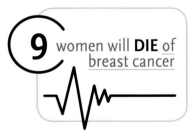

— 2500 women followed for 10 years —

HOW SHOULD YOU DECIDE?

Use this information and combine it with your own values and preferences. There is no "right" answer.

The best decision is the one that feels most comfortable for you.

THOUGHT QUESTIONS

- How important is it to *you* to avoid testing and treatments that are possibly unnecessary?

- How much burden (extra testing and risk of being unnecessarily tested and treated) are *you* willing to accept to improve your chances regarding breast cancer?

- If you think you want to be screened for breast cancer, at what age would *you* like to begin?

- How often would *you* like to have a mammogram?

Ask your health care provider to clarify any questions you may have.

Discuss with friends and family if you like.

Breast Cancer Screening

FOR WOMEN IN THEIR 50s

Clinician Talking Points & Discussion Guide

Below, please find suggested questions and talking points to help guide your conversation with your patient.
If a bullet has a ★ next to it, we <u>highly recommend</u> including this in your discussion.

Introduction

Ask:

★ "Is this a good time for you to discuss breast cancer screening?"

• "Is there anyone else you would like to participate in the conversation, such as a family member?"

Set the Stage

Share:

★ Each chart shows 10,000 women and what happens to them over 10 years based on whether they choose regular mammograms or not.

★ *Explain the meaning of the different color dots:*
  • Green: cancer with good outcome
  • Black: Cancer that causes death

• Though not shown in the charts, in these groups of 10,000 women, there are other cases of breast cancer — some diagnosed and some not — that do not cause death.

Review ANNUAL SCREENING vs. NO SCREENING

Share:

★ There is **no all-cause mortality benefit** from screening mammograms.

• The <u>breast cancer mortality benefit</u> from screening mammograms is **surprisingly small**:
  • Only 1 in 1299 for women in their 50s
  • This is approximated in the chart as 8 in 10,000 women who avoid dying of breast cancer due to having screening mammograms.

★ This benefit —small as it is — comes with harms and risk:
  • The burdens of testing (physical pain, anxiety, inconvenience)
  • The risk of false positives (leading to repeat mammograms or ultrasound +/- biopsies)
  • The risk of overdiagnosis (unnecessary painful, disruptive, disfiguring, costly treatments)

Emphasize:

★ Each dot represents 1 woman, and each chart shows what happens to 10,000 women.

★ **You have an equal chance of being any one of the 10,000 dots.** Your choice is about whether you want to be in the group on the left or the group on the right.

• The left side shows a group of 10,000 women who choose annual mammograms.
  • In this group, there will be 46 women who will be diagnosed with breast cancer in their 50s and eventually die of breast cancer.
  • Because of mammograms, 8 out of 10,000 women avoid this.

• On the right side we see 10,000 women who choose to NOT have mammograms.
  • 54 of these women will be diagnosed with breast cancer in their 50s and eventually die of breast cancer.

★ Having a screening mammogram should be a personal choice because it involves <u>trade-offs among these benefits and harms</u>.

• It is <u>up to **you**</u> to decide based on your values and preferences.

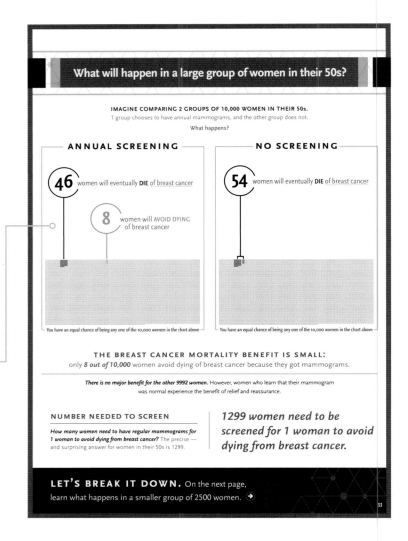

Data for chart adapted from Nelson HD, Cantor A, Humphrey L, Fu R, Pappas M, Daeges M, Griffin J. Screening for Breast Cancer: A Systematic Review to Update the 2009 U.S. Preventive Services Task Force Recommendation. Evidence Synthesis No. 124. *AHRQ* Publication No. 14-05201-EF-1. Rockville, MD: Agency for Healthcare Research and Quality; 2016.

What will happen in a large group of women in their 50s?

IMAGINE COMPARING 2 GROUPS OF 10,000 WOMEN IN THEIR 50s.
1 group chooses to have annual mammograms, and the other group does not.

What happens?

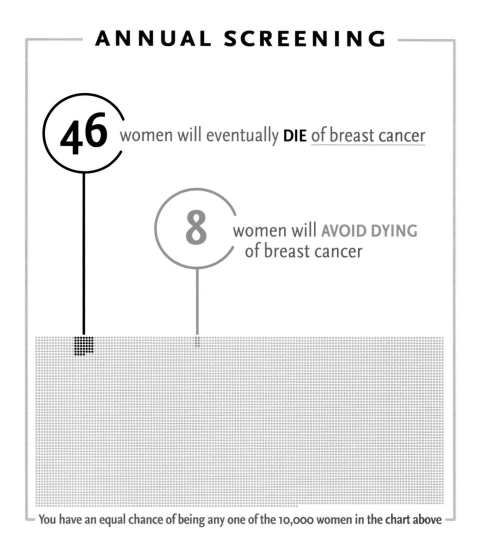

ANNUAL SCREENING

46 women will eventually **DIE** of breast cancer

8 women will **AVOID DYING** of breast cancer

You have an equal chance of being any one of the 10,000 women in the chart above

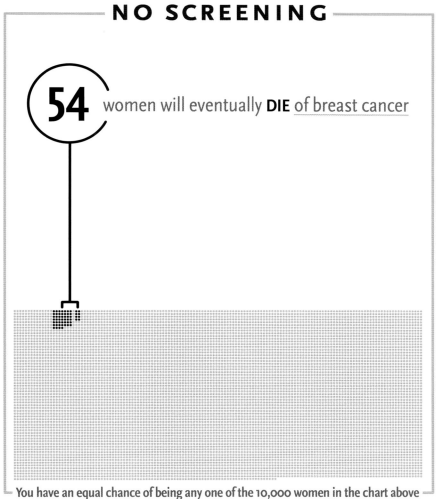

NO SCREENING

54 women will eventually **DIE** of breast cancer

You have an equal chance of being any one of the 10,000 women in the chart above

THE BREAST CANCER MORTALITY BENEFIT IS SMALL:

only **8 out of 10,000** women avoid dying of breast cancer because they got mammograms.

There is no major benefit for the other 9992 women. However, women who learn that their mammogram was normal experience the benefit of relief and reassurance.

NUMBER NEEDED TO SCREEN

How many women need to have regular mammograms for 1 woman to avoid dying from breast cancer? The precise — and surprising answer for women in their 50s is 1299.

1299 women need to be screened for 1 woman to avoid dying from breast cancer.

LET'S BREAK IT DOWN. On the next page,

learn what happens in a smaller group of 2500 women.

Set the Stage

Share:

★ These charts show a little more of what happens to a group of women who choose regular mammograms. This time, we are looking at **2 groups of 2500 women**.

• The group on the left has chosen to <u>have</u> regular screening mammograms.

• The group on the right has chosen to <u>not</u> have regular screening mammograms.

★ Each dot represents 1 woman.

★ You have an **equal chance** of being any one of the women represented by the 2500 dots.

★ In **each** group of 2500 women, 2442 women will not have or get breast cancer, and 58 (43 + 15) will have or get breast cancer.

★ **15 of the 58 breast cancers are turtle-type cancers:** they will not be diagnosed in the No Screening group — and they will never cause any symptoms or harm for those 15 women.

Review the ANNUAL SCREENING Section

• Among the 2442 women without breast cancer, the 909 gray dots (37%) represent women who will have consistently negative mammograms.

★ The 1533 yellow dots (63%) represent women who will have false positive mammograms.

★ **Explain the false positives**: things that are seen on the mammogram that raise a concern of a problem, but after further testing we learn that it was really nothing.

    ★ All 1533 of these women get extra testing; for most of them it is additional imaging tests, such as focused mammogram views or ultrasounds, but:

        ★ **235 will have a biopsy** (a surgical procedure to remove a sample of the breast to examine it under a microscope).

★ Among the 43 women with bad cancers (bears and grenades), the 31 green dots represent women who will **survive** and the **12 black dots** represent women who will **die** of breast cancer. <u>This is the prime benefit of screening, because 2 fewer women die</u> compared to the No Screening group.

★ The **15 red dots represent cases of overdiagnosed breast cancers:** <u>turtle-type cancers that were found only because of the screening</u>.

    • Because these never would have caused symptoms or harm, there is <u>no possible benefit from diagnosing or treating them</u>. Cancer treatments always cause harms. These women will die from something other than breast cancer.

★ **REMEMBER:** At the time of choosing screening, you have an <u>equal chance of being any of the women represented by these 2500 dots</u>.

Review the NO SCREENING Section

• The 2442 gray dots represent the women who do not have or get breast cancer. They have no testing and no problems.

• There are 43 women who will have or get a bad breast cancer (bear- and grenade-type). After developing symptoms, such as a lump, they will get diagnosed with and treated for breast cancer.

    • The 29 green dots represent women who will survive

    • The **14 black dots** represent women who will **die** of breast cancer, **2 more than in the screened group**

★ The 15 green dots **in their own section represent turtle-type cancers**, which will never cause any symptoms or harm. Because there is no screening in this group, they will never be found, so <u>these 15 women will not be harmed by unnecessary treatments</u>.

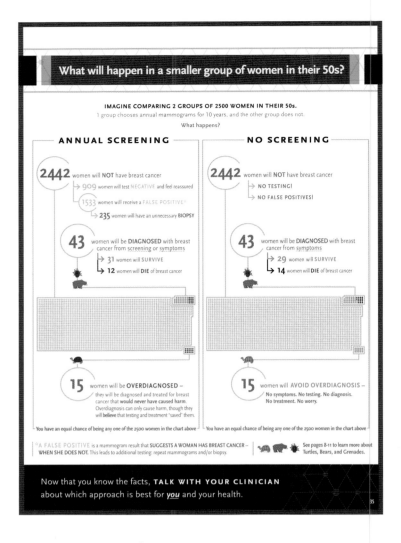

Comments on the Data

• For clarity of presentation, some numbers have been rounded.

• If screening is done <u>every other year</u>, there would be <u>fewer</u> false positives (1050) and unnecessary biopsies (160). See page 37.

• Rates of overdiagnosis have been reported over a wide range (0 – 54%), and the precise rate is not known. Evidence from the best designed studies suggest that at least 20% of screen-detected breast cancers represent overdiagnosis.[1,2,3] In this book, a rate of 25% has been assumed.

Data for chart adapted from:

Nelson HD, Cantor A, Humphrey L, Fu R, Pappas M, Daeges M, Griffin J. Screening for Breast Cancer: A Systematic Review to Update the 2009 U.S. Preventive Services Task Force Recommendation. Evidence Synthesis No. 124. *AHRQ* Publication No. 14-05201-EF-1. Rockville, MD: Agency for Healthcare Research and Quality; 2016.

Howlader N, Noone AM, Krapcho M, Miller D, Bishop K, Kosary CL, Yu M, Ruhl J, Tatalovich Z, Mariotto A, Lewis DR, Chen HS, Feuer EJ, Cronin KA (eds). *SEER Cancer Statistics Review*, 1975-2014, National Cancer Institute. Bethesda, MD, https://seer.cancer.gov/csr/1975_2014/, based on November 2016 SEER data submission, posted to the SEER web site, April 2017.

Hubbard RA, Kerlikowske K, Flowers CI, et al. Cumulative probability of false-positive recall or biopsy recommendation after 10 years of screening mammography: a cohort study. *Ann Intern Med*. 2011;155(8): 481-92. PMID: 22007042.

1. Bleyer A, Welch HG: Effect of three decades of screening mammography on breast-cancer incidence. *N Engl J Med* 367 (21): 1998-2005, 2012.

2. Kalager M, Zelen M, Langmark F, et al.: Effect of screening mammography on breast-cancer mortality in Norway. *N Engl J Med* 363 (13): 1203-10, 2010.

3. Jørgensen KJ, Gøtzsche PC: Overdiagnosis in publicly organised mammography screening programmes: systematic review of incidence trends. *BMJ* 339: b2587, 2009.

IMAGINE COMPARING 2 GROUPS OF 2500 WOMEN IN THEIR 50s.

1 group chooses annual mammograms for 10 years, and the other group does not.

What happens?

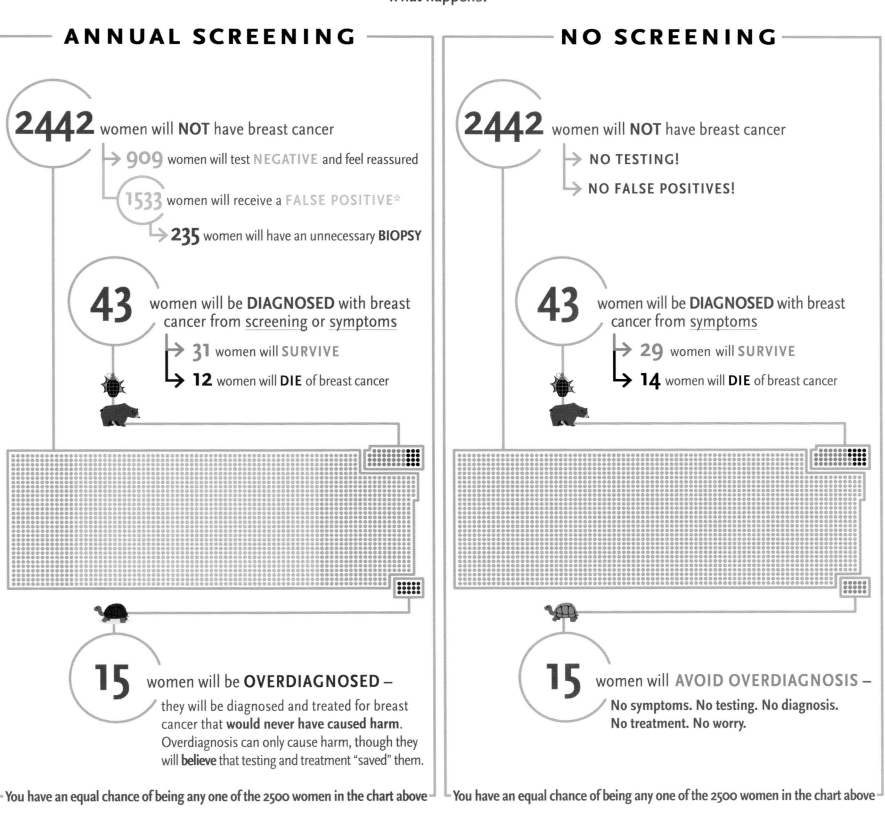

ANNUAL SCREENING

2442 women will **NOT** have breast cancer

→ **909** women will test NEGATIVE and feel reassured

1533 women will receive a FALSE POSITIVE*

→ **235** women will have an unnecessary **BIOPSY**

43 women will be **DIAGNOSED** with breast cancer from <u>screening</u> or <u>symptoms</u>

→ **31** women will SURVIVE

→ **12** women will **DIE** of breast cancer

15 women will be **OVERDIAGNOSED** –

they will be diagnosed and treated for breast cancer that **would never have caused harm**. Overdiagnosis can only cause harm, though they will **believe** that testing and treatment "saved" them.

You have an equal chance of being any one of the 2500 women in the chart above

NO SCREENING

2442 women will **NOT** have breast cancer

→ **NO TESTING!**

→ **NO FALSE POSITIVES!**

43 women will be **DIAGNOSED** with breast cancer from <u>symptoms</u>

→ **29** women will SURVIVE

→ **14** women will **DIE** of breast cancer

15 women will AVOID OVERDIAGNOSIS –

No symptoms. No testing. No diagnosis. No treatment. No worry.

You have an equal chance of being any one of the 2500 women in the chart above

---

*A FALSE POSITIVE is a mammogram result that **SUGGESTS A WOMAN HAS BREAST CANCER – WHEN SHE DOES NOT.** This leads to additional testing: repeat mammograms and/or biopsy.

 See pages 8-11 to learn more about Turtles, Bears, and Grenades.

Now that you know the facts, **TALK WITH YOUR CLINICIAN** about which approach is best for **you** and your health.

Set the Stage

Share:

- This page helps you compare 3 different strategies or approaches. The numbers show what happens to 3 groups of 2500 women in their 50s.

★ "As we look at these, consider which one feels most appropriate FOR YOU. **I am happy to support whatever choice you make.**"

Review the REGULAR SCREENING Section

Share:

- The first 2 rows show the outcomes for women who choose screening mammograms.
  - In the first row, women are getting a mammogram <u>every year</u>.
  - In the second row, women are getting a mammogram <u>every other year</u>.

★ The main differences are <u>fewer false positives and biopsies</u> in the group that has mammograms every other year.

Review the NO SCREENING Section

Share:

- In the last row, we see what happens to 2500 women who choose to not have screening mammograms.

★ You can see that they avoid false positives, unnecessary biopsies, and overdiagnosed cases of breast cancer, but <u>2 more women die of breast cancer in this group</u>.

- This is just 1 extra breast cancer death **per 2500 women**, and

- There is **no difference in all-cause mortality**.

Emphasize:

★ When considering whether you want a screening mammogram, there is no one "right" answer.

★ **The best decision is the one that feels most comfortable to <u>you</u>.**

Review the HOW SHOULD YOU DECIDE? Section

Share:

★ You might find it helpful to consider some of these questions.

Ask:

- Do you have any questions for me?
- Do you feel ready to make a decision?

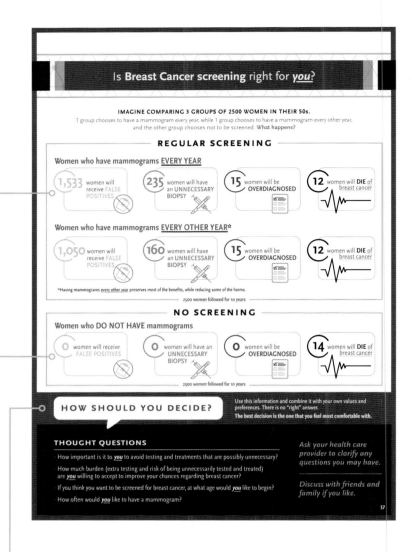

Did you know? *False positive rates are > 20% higher in obese women[1].*

1. Elmore JG, Carney PA, Abraham LA, et al.: The association between obesity and screening mammography accuracy. Arch Intern Med 164 (10): 1140-7, 2004

Is **Breast Cancer screening** right for *you*?

IMAGINE COMPARING 3 GROUPS OF 2500 WOMEN IN THEIR 50s.

1 group chooses to have a mammogram every year, while 1 group chooses to have a mammogram every other year, and the other group chooses not to be screened. **What happens?**

REGULAR SCREENING

Women who have mammograms EVERY YEAR

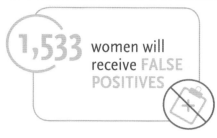

1,533 women will receive FALSE POSITIVES

235 women will have an UNNECESSARY BIOPSY

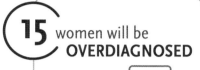

15 women will be OVERDIAGNOSED

12 women will **DIE** of breast cancer

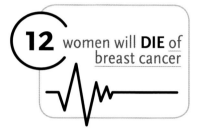

Women who have mammograms EVERY OTHER YEAR*

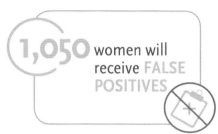

1,050 women will receive FALSE POSITIVES

160 women will have an UNNECESSARY BIOPSY

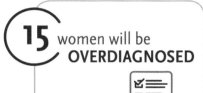

15 women will be OVERDIAGNOSED

12 women will **DIE** of breast cancer

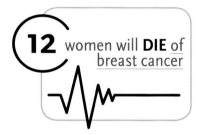

*Having mammograms <u>every other year</u> preserves most of the benefits, while reducing some of the harms.

— 2500 women followed for 10 years —

NO SCREENING

Women who DO NOT HAVE mammograms

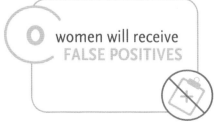

0 women will receive FALSE POSITIVES

0 women will have an UNNECESSARY BIOPSY

0 women will be OVERDIAGNOSED

14 women will **DIE** of breast cancer

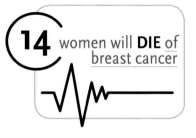

— 2500 women followed for 10 years —

HOW SHOULD YOU DECIDE?

Use this information and combine it with your own values and preferences. There is no "right" answer.

The best decision is the one that you feel most comfortable with.

THOUGHT QUESTIONS

- How important is it to *you* to avoid testing and treatments that are possibly unnecessary?

- How much burden (extra testing and risk of being unnecessarily tested and treated) are *you* willing to accept to improve your chances regarding breast cancer?

- If you think you want to be screened for breast cancer, at what age would *you* like to begin?

- How often would *you* like to have a mammogram?

Ask your health care provider to clarify any questions you may have.

Discuss with friends and family if you like.

37

Breast Cancer Screening

FOR WOMEN IN THEIR 60s

Clinician Talking Points & Discussion Guide

Below, please find suggested questions and talking points to help guide your conversation with your patient.
If a bullet has a ★ next to it, we <u>highly recommend</u> including this in your discussion.

Introduction

Ask:

★ "Is this a good time for you to discuss breast cancer screening?"

• "Is there anyone else you would like to participate in the conversation, such as a family member?"

Set the Stage

Share:

★ Each chart shows 10,000 women and what happens to them over 10 years based on whether they choose regular mammograms or not.

★ *Explain the meaning of the different color dots:*
  • Green: cancer with good outcome
  • Black: Cancer that causes death

• Though not shown in the charts, in these groups of 10,000 women, there are other cases of breast cancer — some diagnosed and some not — that do not cause death.

Review ANNUAL SCREENING vs. NO SCREENING

Share:

★ There is **no all-cause mortality benefit** from screening mammograms.

• The <u>breast cancer mortality benefit</u> from screening mammograms is **surprisingly small:**
  • Only 1 in 469 for women in their 60s
  • This is approximated in the chart as 21 in 10,000 women who avoid dying of breast cancer due to having screening mammograms.

★ This benefit —small as it is — comes with harms and risk:
  • The burdens of testing (physical pain, anxiety, inconvenience)
  • The risk of false positives (leading to repeat mammograms or ultrasound +/- biopsies)
  • The risk of overdiagnosis (unnecessary painful, disruptive, disfiguring, costly treatments)

Emphasize:

★ Each dot represents 1 woman, and each chart shows what happens to 10,000 women.

★ **You have an equal chance of being any one of the 10,000 dots.** Your choice is about whether you want to be in the group on the left or the group on the right.

• The left side shows a group of 10,000 women who choose annual mammograms.
  • In this group, there will be 44 women who will be diagnosed with breast cancer in their 60s and eventually die of breast cancer.
  • Because of mammograms, 21 out of 10,000 women avoid this.

• On the right side we see 10,000 women who choose to NOT have mammograms.
  • 65 of these women will be diagnosed with breast cancer in their 60s and eventually die of breast cancer.

★ Having a screening mammogram should be a personal choice because it involves <u>trade-offs among these benefits and harms.</u>

• It is <u>up to **you**</u> to decide based on your values and preferences.

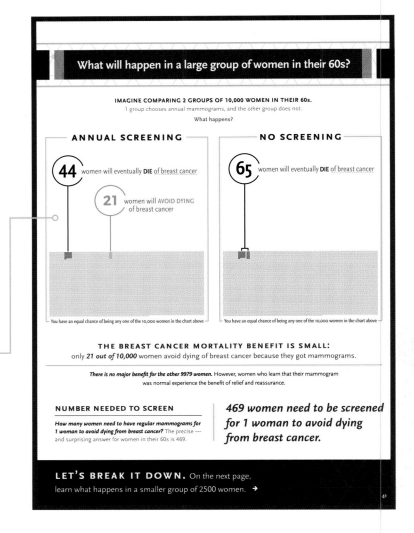

Data for chart adapted from Nelson HD, Cantor A, Humphrey L, Fu R, Pappas M, Daeges M, Griffin J. Screening for Breast Cancer: A Systematic Review to Update the 2009 U.S. Preventive Services Task Force Recommendation. Evidence Synthesis No. 124. *AHRQ* Publication No. 14-05201-EF-1. Rockville, MD: Agency for Healthcare Research and Quality; 2016.

What will happen in a large group of women in their 60s?

IMAGINE COMPARING 2 GROUPS OF 10,000 WOMEN IN THEIR 60s.

1 group chooses annual mammograms, and the other group does not.

What happens?

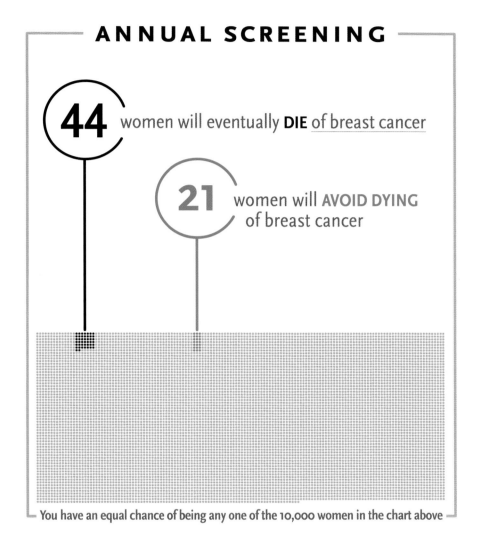

ANNUAL SCREENING

44 women will eventually **DIE** of breast cancer

21 women will **AVOID DYING** of breast cancer

You have an equal chance of being any one of the 10,000 women in the chart above

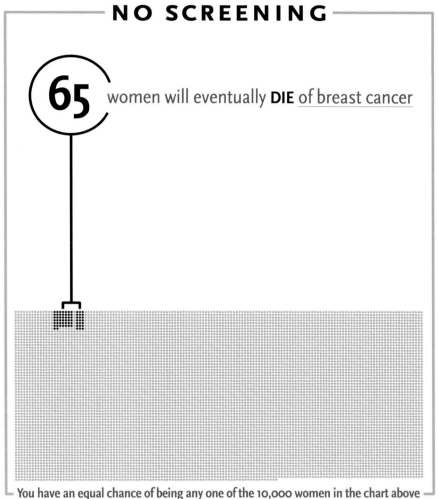

NO SCREENING

65 women will eventually **DIE** of breast cancer

You have an equal chance of being any one of the 10,000 women in the chart above

THE BREAST CANCER MORTALITY BENEFIT IS SMALL:

only *21 out of 10,000* women avoid dying of breast cancer because they got mammograms.

There is no major benefit for the other 9979 women. However, women who learn that their mammogram was normal experience the benefit of relief and reassurance.

NUMBER NEEDED TO SCREEN

How many women need to have regular mammograms for 1 woman to avoid dying from breast cancer? The precise — and surprising answer for women in their 60s is 469.

469 women need to be screened for 1 woman to avoid dying from breast cancer.

Set the Stage

Share:

★ These charts show a little more of what happens to a group of women who choose regular mammograms. This time, we are looking at **2 groups of 2500 women.**

• The group on the left has chosen to <u>have</u> regular screening mammograms.

• The group on the right has chosen to <u>not</u> have regular screening mammograms.

★ Each dot represents 1 woman.

★ You have an **equal chance** of being any one of the women represented by the 2500 dots.

★ In **each** group of 2500 women, 2412 women will not have or get breast cancer, and 86 (64 + 22) will have or get breast cancer.

★ **22 of the 86 breast cancers are turtle-type cancers:** they will not be diagnosed in the No Screening group — and they will never cause any symptoms or harm for those 22 women.

Review the ANNUAL SCREENING Section

• Among the 2414 women without breast cancer, the 1174 gray dots (49%) represent women who will have consistently negative mammograms.

★ The 1240 yellow dots (51%) represent women who will have false positive mammograms.

★ **Explain the false positives:** things that are seen on the mammogram that raise a concern of a problem, but after further testing we learn that it was really nothing.

   ★ All 1240 of these women get extra testing; for most of them it is additional imaging tests, such as focused mammogram views or ultrasounds, but:

     ★ **175 will have a biopsy** (a surgical procedure to remove a sample of the breast to examine it under a microscope).

★ Among the 64 women with bad cancers (bears and grenades), the 53 green dots represent women who will **survive** and the **11 black dots** represent women who will **die** of breast cancer. <u>This is the prime benefit of screening, because 5 fewer women die</u> compared to the No Screening group.

★ The **22 red dots represent cases of overdiagnosed breast cancers:** <u>turtle-type cancers that were found only because of the screening.</u>

   • Because these never would have caused symptoms or harm, there is <u>no possible benefit from diagnosing or treating them</u>. Cancer treatments always cause harms. These women will die from something other than breast cancer.

★ **REMEMBER:** At the time of choosing screening, you have an <u>equal chance of being any of the women represented by these 2500 dots.</u>

Review the NO SCREENING Section

• The 2414 gray dots represent the women who do not have or get breast cancer. They have no testing and no problems.

• There are 64 women who will have or get a bad breast cancer (bear- and grenade-type). After developing symptoms, such as a lump, they will get diagnosed with and treated for breast cancer.

   • The 48 green dots represent women who will survive

   • The **16 black dots** represent women who will **die** of breast cancer, **5 more than in the screened group**

★ The 22 green dots **in their own section represent turtle-type cancers**, which will never cause any symptoms or harm. Because there is no screening in this group, they will never be found, so <u>these 22 women will not be harmed by unnecessary treatments.</u>

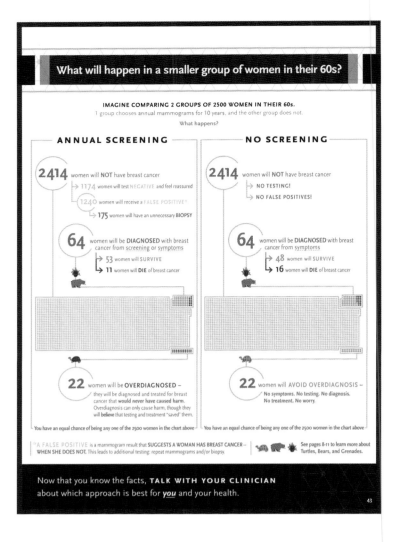

Comments on the Data

• For clarity of presentation, some numbers have been rounded.

• If screening is done <u>every other year</u>, there would be <u>fewer</u> false positives (850) <u>and unnecessary biopsies (120)</u>. See page 45.

• Rates of overdiagnosis have been reported over a wide range (0 – 54%), and the precise rate is not known. Evidence from the best designed studies suggest that at least 20% of screen-detected breast cancers represent overdiagnosis.[1,2,3] In this book, a rate of 25% has been assumed.

Data for chart adapted from:

Nelson HD, Cantor A, Humphrey L, Fu R, Pappas M, Daeges M, Griffin J. Screening for Breast Cancer: A Systematic Review to Update the 2009 U.S. Preventive Services Task Force Recommendation. Evidence Synthesis No. 124. *AHRQ* Publication No. 14-05201-EF-1. Rockville, MD: Agency for Healthcare Research and Quality; 2016.

Howlader N, Noone AM, Krapcho M, Miller D, Bishop K, Kosary CL, Yu M, Ruhl J, Tatalovich Z, Mariotto A, Lewis DR, Chen HS, Feuer EJ, Cronin KA (eds). *SEER Cancer Statistics Review*, 1975-2014, National Cancer Institute. Bethesda, MD, https://seer.cancer.gov/csr/1975_2014/, based on November 2016 SEER data submission, posted to the SEER web site, April 2017.

Hubbard RA, Kerlikowske K, Flowers CI, et al. Cumulative probability of false-positive recall or biopsy recommendation after 10 years of screening mammography: a cohort study. *Ann Intern Med.* 2011;155(8): 481-92. PMID: 22007042.

1. Bleyer A, Welch HG: Effect of three decades of screening mammography on breast-cancer incidence. *N Engl J Med* 367 (21): 1998-2005, 2012.

2. Kalager M, Zelen M, Langmark F, et al.: Effect of screening mammography on breast-cancer mortality in Norway. *N Engl J Med* 363 (13): 1203-10, 2010.

3. Jørgensen KJ, Gøtzsche PC: Overdiagnosis in publicly organised mammography screening programmes: systematic review of incidence trends. *BMJ* 339: b2587, 2009.

What will happen in a smaller group of women in their 60s?

IMAGINE COMPARING 2 GROUPS OF 2500 WOMEN IN THEIR 60s.

1 group chooses annual mammograms for 10 years, and the other group does not.

What happens?

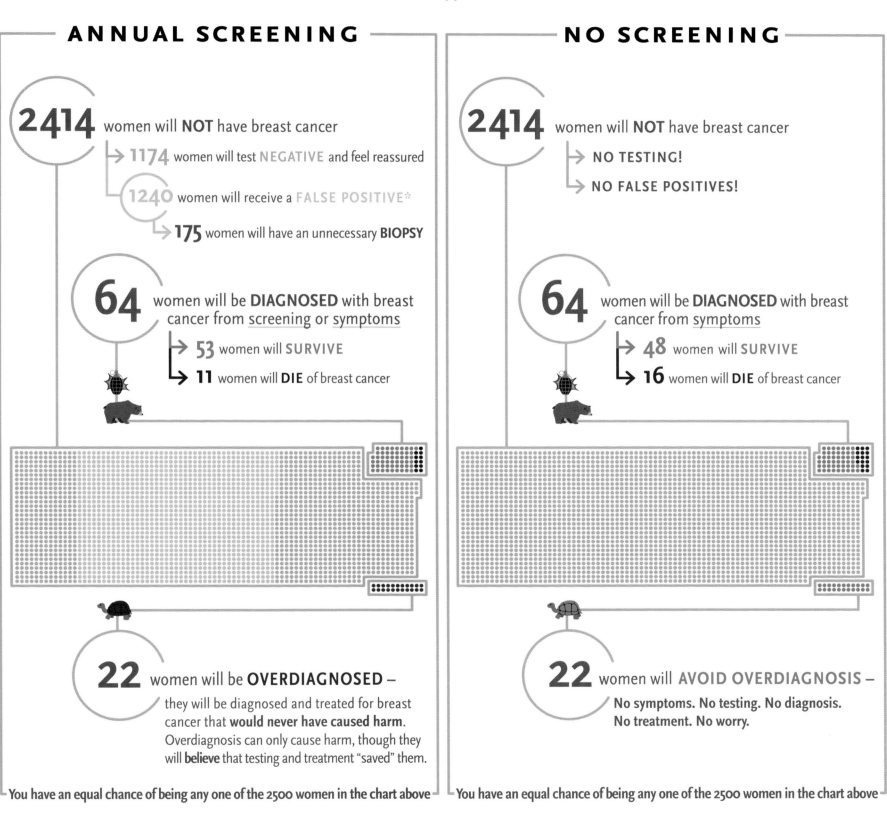

ANNUAL SCREENING

2414 women will **NOT** have breast cancer

→ **1174** women will test NEGATIVE and feel reassured

1240 women will receive a FALSE POSITIVE*

→ **175** women will have an unnecessary **BIOPSY**

64 women will be **DIAGNOSED** with breast cancer from <u>screening</u> or <u>symptoms</u>

→ **53** women will SURVIVE

→ **11** women will **DIE** of breast cancer

22 women will be **OVERDIAGNOSED** –
they will be diagnosed and treated for breast cancer that **would never have caused harm**. Overdiagnosis can only cause harm, though they will **believe** that testing and treatment "saved" them.

You have an equal chance of being any one of the 2500 women in the chart above

NO SCREENING

2414 women will **NOT** have breast cancer

→ **NO TESTING!**

→ **NO FALSE POSITIVES!**

64 women will be **DIAGNOSED** with breast cancer from <u>symptoms</u>

→ **48** women will SURVIVE

→ **16** women will **DIE** of breast cancer

22 women will AVOID OVERDIAGNOSIS –
No symptoms. No testing. No diagnosis. No treatment. No worry.

You have an equal chance of being any one of the 2500 women in the chart above

---

*A FALSE POSITIVE is a mammogram result that **SUGGESTS A WOMAN HAS BREAST CANCER – WHEN SHE DOES NOT.** This leads to additional testing: repeat mammograms and/or biopsy.

 See pages 8-11 to learn more about Turtles, Bears, and Grenades.

Set the Stage

Share:

- This page helps you compare 3 different strategies or approaches. The numbers show what happens to 3 groups of 2500 women in their 50s.

★ "As we look at these, consider which one feels most appropriate FOR YOU. **I am happy to support whatever choice you make.**"

Review the REGULAR SCREENING Section

Share:

- The first 2 rows show the outcomes for women who choose screening mammograms.
  - In the first row, women are getting a mammogram <u>every year</u>.
  - In the second row, women are getting a mammogram <u>every other year</u>.

★ The main differences are <u>fewer false positives and biopsies</u> in the group that has mammograms every other year.

Review the NO SCREENING Section

Share:

- In the last row, we see what happens to 2500 women who choose to not have screening mammograms.

★ You can see that they avoid false positives, unnecessary biopsies, and overdiagnosed cases of breast cancer, but <u>5 more women die of breast cancer in this group</u>.

- This is just 1 extra breast cancer death **per 2500 women**, and

- There is **no difference in all-cause mortality**.

Emphasize:

★ When considering whether you want a screening mammogram, there is no one "right" answer.

★ **The best decision is the one that feels most comfortable to <u>you</u>.**

Review the HOW SHOULD YOU DECIDE? Section

Share:

★ You might find it helpful to consider some of these questions.

Ask:

- Do you have any questions for me?
- Do you feel ready to make a decision?

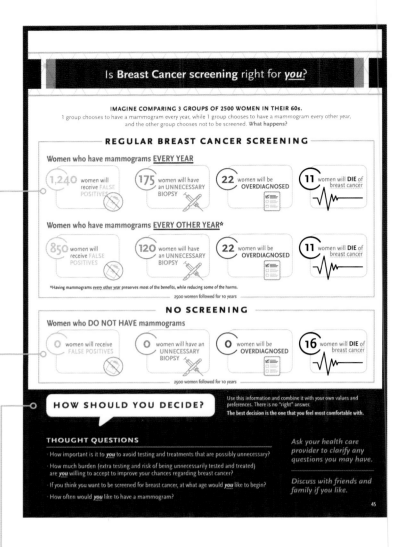

Did you know? *False positive rates are > 20% higher in obese women[1].*

1. Elmore JG, Carney PA, Abraham LA, et al.: The association between obesity and screening mammography accuracy. Arch Intern Med 164 (10): 1140-7, 2004

Is **Breast Cancer screening** right for *you*?

IMAGINE COMPARING 3 GROUPS OF 2500 WOMEN IN THEIR 60s.

1 group chooses to have a mammogram every year, while 1 group chooses to have a mammogram every other year, and the other group chooses not to be screened. **What happens?**

REGULAR BREAST CANCER SCREENING

Women who have mammograms EVERY YEAR

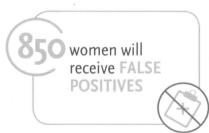 **1,240** women will receive FALSE POSITIVES

175 women will have an UNNECESSARY BIOPSY

22 women will be OVERDIAGNOSED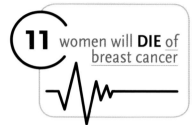

11 women will **DIE** of breast cancer

Women who have mammograms EVERY OTHER YEAR✳

850 women will receive FALSE POSITIVES

120 women will have an UNNECESSARY BIOPSY

22 women will be OVERDIAGNOSED

11 women will **DIE** of breast cancer

*Having mammograms <u>every other year</u> preserves most of the benefits, while reducing some of the harms.

— 2500 women followed for 10 years —

NO SCREENING

Women who DO NOT HAVE mammograms

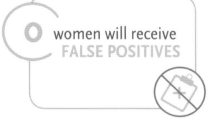 **0** women will receive FALSE POSITIVES

0 women will have an UNNECESSARY BIOPSY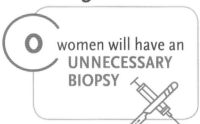

0 women will be OVERDIAGNOSED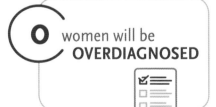

16 women will **DIE** of breast cancer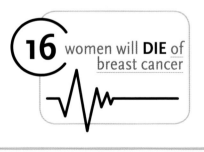

— 2500 women followed for 10 years —

HOW SHOULD YOU DECIDE?

Use this information and combine it with your own values and preferences. There is no "right" answer.

The best decision is the one that you feel most comfortable with.

THOUGHT QUESTIONS

- How important is it to *you* to avoid testing and treatments that are possibly unnecessary?

- How much burden (extra testing and risk of being unnecessarily tested and treated) are *you* willing to accept to improve your chances regarding breast cancer?

- If you think you want to be screened for breast cancer, at what age would *you* like to begin?

Ask your health care provider to clarify any questions you may have.

Discuss with friends and family if you like.

Colorectal Cancer Screening

Clinician Talking Points & Discussion Guide

Below, please find suggested questions and talking points to help guide your conversation with your patient.
If a bullet has a ★ next to it, we <u>highly recommend</u> including this in your discussion.

Introduction

Ask:

★ "Is this a good time for you to discuss colorectal cancer screening?"

• "Is there anyone else you would like to participate in the conversation, such as a family member?"

Share:

★ While screening is recommended for everyone age 50-75 years, <u>patients can choose between 2 main methods of screening</u>: colonoscopy or a stool test (FIT) that they can do at home.

Review | WHY WOULD I WANT TO GET SCREENED?

Share:

★ **Risk increases with age**.

• CRC is most frequently diagnosed among people age 65-74 years. Median age at death: 68.

★ CRC arises from a polyp, and we have tests that can help find these.

★ Screening is useful because it takes a long time for a polyp to progress to cancer.

• Not all polyps are pre-cancerous.

Review | If I choose CRC screening, WHAT IS THE BEST TEST FOR ME?

Describe the 2 primary testing options: FIT and Colonoscopy

Share:

★ "Both options are reasonable. The choice is yours, and it involves trade-offs among factors such as comfort, convenience, cost, and thoroughness."

★ "My patients rarely complain about pain with the colonoscopy, but they do sometimes complain about the prep the day before, which will involve a lot of time in the bathroom."

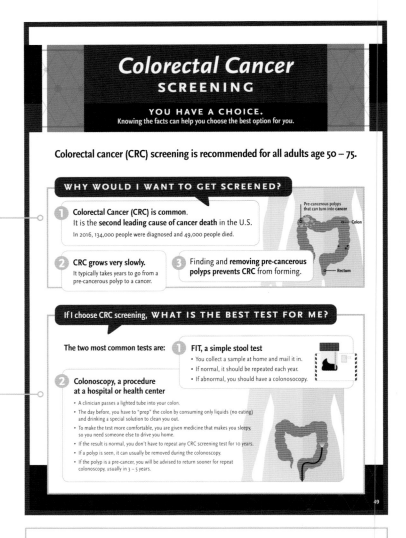

CRC Screening Effect on Overall Mortality

★ Though CRC screening has been shown to reduce mortality from CRC, it has not been shown to reduce overall or all-cause mortality.[4]

Additional Information

• **Some patients may inquire about other screening tests, especially CT colonography**. This is <u>less effective</u> and <u>more costly</u> than FIT or colonoscopy. It requires the same bowel prep as colonoscopy, but does not allow for polypectomy; patients with polyps identified would need to return for colonoscopy. If negative, it should be repeated every 5 years.

• About 1/3 of eligible adults have never been screened for CRC.[1,2]

• Evidence suggests that screening rates rise when patients are offered a choice regarding screening tests.[3]

★ **The best test is the one that gets done.**

USPSTF Recommendation:[5]

• The USPSTF recommends screening for colorectal cancer starting at age 50 years and continuing until age 75 years.

• The decision to screen for colorectal cancer in adults aged 76 to 85 years should be an individual one, taking into account the patient's overall health and prior screening history.

• **N.B. The information above is for people without symptoms who are at average risk for CRC and who do not have a family history of known genetic disorders that predispose them to a high lifetime risk of colorectal cancer** (such as Lynch syndrome or familial adenomatous polyposis), a personal history of inflammatory bowel disease, a previous adenomatous polyp, or previous colorectal cancer. When screening results in the diagnosis of colorectal adenomas or cancer, patients are followed up with a surveillance regimen, and recommendations for screening no longer apply.

• **A positive family history (excluding known inherited familial syndromes) is thought to be linked to about 20% of cases of colorectal cancer.** About 3% to 10% of the population has a first-degree relative with colorectal cancer. The USPSTF did not specifically review the evidence on screening in populations at increased risk; however, other professional organizations recommend that patients with a family history of colorectal cancer (a first-degree relative with early onset colorectal cancer or multiple first-degree relatives with the disease) be screened more frequently starting at a younger age and with colonoscopy. Patients with a first degree relative who had CRC diagnosed before age 60, should begin screening earlier: age 40 or 10 years earlier than the age at which the relative was diagnosed, whichever is earlier. Male sex and black race are also associated with higher colorectal cancer incidence and mortality.

1. Shapiro JA, Klabunde CN, Thompson TD, Nadel MR, Seeff LC, White A. Patterns of colorectal cancer test use, including CT colonography, in the 2010 National Health Interview Survey. *Cancer Epidemiol Biomarkers Prev.* 2012;21(6):895-904.

2. Centers for Disease Control and Prevention (CDC). Vital signs: colorectal cancer screening test use: United States, 2012. *MMWR Morb Mortal Wkly Rep.* 2013;62(44):881-888.

3. Inadomi JM, Vijan S, Janz NK, et al. Adherence to colorectal cancer screening: a randomized clinical trial of competing strategies. *Arch Intern Med.* 2012;172(7):575-582.

4. Shaukat A, Mongin SJ, Geisser MS, et al. Long-term mortality after screening for colorectal cancer. *N Engl J Med* 2013; 369:1106-14.

5. U.S. Preventive Services Task Force, Bibbins-Domingo K, Grossman DC, et al. Screening for colorectal cancer: US Preventive Services Task Force recommendation statement. *JAMA* 2016; 315: 2564-75.

Colorectal Cancer
SCREENING

YOU HAVE A CHOICE.
Knowing the facts can help you choose the best option for you.

Colorectal cancer (CRC) screening is recommended for all adults age 50 – 75.

WHY WOULD I WANT TO GET SCREENED?

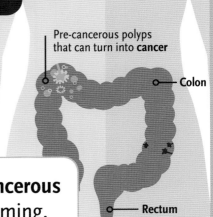

Pre-cancerous polyps that can turn into **cancer**

Colon

Rectum

1 **Colorectal Cancer (CRC) is common.**
It is the **second leading cause of cancer death** in the U.S.

In 2016, 134,000 people were diagnosed and 49,000 people died.

2 **CRC grows very slowly.**
It typically takes years to go from a pre-cancerous polyp to a cancer.

3 Finding and **removing pre-cancerous polyps prevents CRC** from forming.

If I choose CRC screening, WHAT IS THE BEST TEST FOR ME?

The two most common tests are:

1 **FIT, a simple stool test**

- You collect a sample at home and mail it in.
- If normal, it should be repeated each year.
- If abnormal, you should have a colonosocopy.

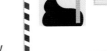

2 **Colonoscopy, a procedure at a hospital or health center**

- A clinician passes a lighted tube into your colon.
- The day before, you have to "prep" the colon by consuming only liquids (no eating) and drinking a special solution to clean you out.
- To make the test more comfortable, you are given medicine that makes you sleepy, so you need someone else to drive you home.
- If the result is normal, you don't have to repeat any CRC screening test for 10 years.
- If a polyp is seen, it can usually be removed during the colonoscopy.
- If the polyp is a pre-cancer, you will be advised to return sooner for repeat colonoscopy, usually in 3 – 5 years.

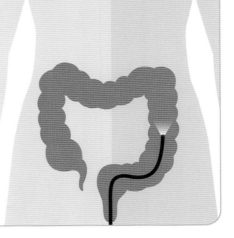

Set the Stage

Share:

★ "To help you assess these trade-offs and make a choice, let's think about 3000 people who are 50 years old, and let's ask 'What happens to them over the next 25 years?'"

★ "Imagine that among these 3000 people, 1000 choose not to have any CRC screening, 1000 choose annual FIT (stool) tests, and 1000 choose colonoscopy every 10 years."

Review the NO SCREENING Section

Share:

★ This section shows what happens to the 1000 people who choose no screening – there are **no screening colonoscopies in this group**.

• The only people who get colonoscopy are those who develop colon symptoms, such as blood in the stool.

★ 70 people get diagnosed with CRC, and 42 survive after treatment (usually surgery, plus other interventions). 28 die of CRC.

Review the CRC SCREENING Section

Share:

• This section compares FIT and colonoscopy.

★ With both screening methods, not only are there fewer CRC deaths, but there are fewer cases of diagnosed CRC, because screening leads to identification and treatment of polyps, which prevents many cancers from forming:

    ★ 70 – 23 = 47 prevented cancers in the FIT group
    ★ 70 – 13 = 57 prevented cancers in the colonoscopy group

Explain more about FIT:

★ Only 5 people out of 1000 die from CRC over 25 years, compared to 28 in the no screening group.

★ Even though this is the FIT group, colonoscopies still happen for some patients: those who have an abnormal FIT result:

    ★ Over 25 years, a group of 1000 people choosing FIT would have a total of 1757 colonoscopies, an average of 1-2 per person.

    • 10 of these people will have a serious complication from their colonoscopy.
        • The risk of colonoscopy complication rises with age.
        • Serious complications may include ileus, bleeding complications, bowel perforation, plus a variety of cardiovascular events, including MI, angina, arrhythmia, CHF, cardiac arrest, syncope, hypotension, and shock.

Explain more about the Colonoscopy group:

★ Because colonoscopy allows for detection and removal of precancerous polyps, there are only 13 cases of CRC in this group.

    ★ Only 4 people die of CRC.
    ★ The trade-off is that this group has more colonoscopies: 4049, or about 4 per person.
        • Some people will have colonoscopies more often than every 10 years to follow up on polyps that were identified.
        • 15 people will have a serious complication (as above) from a colonoscopy.

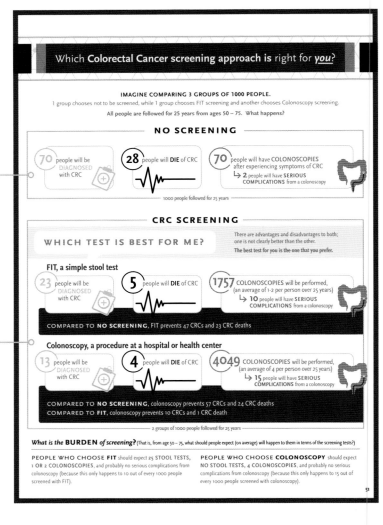

Summary

★ Make sure the patient sees the sections in blue that compare the different strategies and the section at the bottom that describes the burdens of screening:

    • Compared to no screening, FIT prevents 47 CRCs and 23 CRC deaths.
    • Compared to no screening, colonoscopy prevents 57 CRCs and 24 CRC deaths.
    • Compared to FIT, colonoscopy prevents 10 CRCs and 1 CRC death.
    • People who choose screening with FIT should expect 1 or 2 lifetime colonoscopies.
    • People who choose screening with colonoscopy should expect about 4 lifetime colonoscopies.

Debrief

State:

★ "We reviewed a lot of information today."

Ask:

• "Are there are any parts of it you would like to go over again?"

★ "Do you have any questions?"

★ "Do you feel ready to make a decision?"

Inadomi JM. Screening for colorectal neoplasia. *New Engl J Med* 2017;376:149-56.

Zauber A, Knudsen A, Rutter CM, Lansdorp-Vogelaar I, Kuntz KM. Evaluating the benefits and harms of colorectal cancer screening strategies: a collaborative modeling approach. Rockville, MD: Agency for Healthcare Research and Quality, October 2015. (AHRQ publication no. 14-05203-EF-2) (https://www.uspreventiveservicestaskforce.org/Home/GetFile/1/16540/cisnet-draft-modeling-report/pdf).

Which **Colorectal Cancer screening approach is** right for **you**?

IMAGINE COMPARING 3 GROUPS OF 1000 PEOPLE.

1 group chooses not to be screened, while 1 group chooses FIT screening and another chooses Colonoscopy screening.

All people are followed for 25 years from ages 50 – 75. What happens?

NO SCREENING

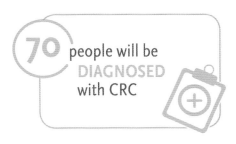 **70** people will be DIAGNOSED with CRC

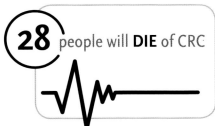 **28** people will **DIE** of CRC

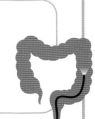 **70** people will have **COLONOSCOPIES** after experiencing symptoms of CRC
↳ **2** people will have **SERIOUS COMPLICATIONS** from a colonoscopy

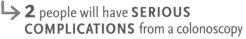

— 1000 people followed for 25 years —

CRC SCREENING

WHICH TEST IS BEST FOR ME?

There are advantages and disadvantages to both; one is not clearly better than the other.

The best test for you is the one that you prefer.

FIT, a simple stool test

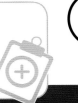 **23** people will be DIAGNOSED with CRC

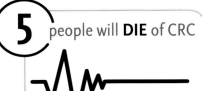 **5** people will **DIE** of CRC

 1757 COLONOSCOPIES will be performed, (an average of 1-2 per person over 25 years)
↳ **10** people will have **SERIOUS COMPLICATIONS** from a colonoscopy

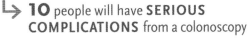

COMPARED TO **NO SCREENING**, FIT prevents 47 CRCs and 23 CRC deaths

Colonoscopy, a procedure at a hospital or health center

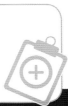 **13** people will be DIAGNOSED with CRC

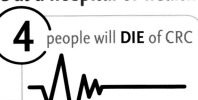 **4** people will **DIE** of CRC

 4049 COLONOSCOPIES will be performed, (an average of 4 per person over 25 years)
↳ **15** people will have **SERIOUS COMPLICATIONS** from a colonoscopy

COMPARED TO **NO SCREENING**, colonoscopy prevents 57 CRCs and 24 CRC deaths
COMPARED TO **FIT**, colonoscopy prevents 10 CRCs and 1 CRC death

— 2 groups of 1000 people followed for 25 years —

What is the BURDEN *of screening?* (That is, from age 50 – 75, what should people expect (on average) will happen to them in terms of the screening tests?)

PEOPLE WHO CHOOSE FIT should expect **25 STOOL TESTS, 1 OR 2 COLONOSCOPIES**, and probably no serious complications from colonoscopy (because this only happens to 10 out of every 1000 people screened with FIT).

PEOPLE WHO CHOOSE COLONOSCOPY should expect **NO STOOL TESTS, 4 COLONOSCOPIES**, and probably no serious complications from colonoscopy (because this only happens to 15 out of every 1000 people screened with colonoscopy).

Lung Cancer Screening

Clinician Talking Points & Discussion Guide

Below, please find suggested questions and talking points to help guide your conversation with your patient.
If a bullet has a ★ next to it, we <u>highly recommend</u> including this in your discussion.

Introduction

Ask:

★ "Is this a good time for you to discuss lung cancer screening?"

• "Is there anyone else you would like to participate in the conversation, such as a family member?"

Review Lung Cancer Screening Eligibility **Section**

★ *Confirm that the patient is eligible.*

• Eligibility:
  • Age 55 – 74 years
  • Smoking history of at least 30 pack-years
  • Still smoking or quit smoking < 15 years ago

Review WHAT IS THE TEST?

Share:

★ The testing is optional, and the patient should decide if s/he wants it based on her/his values and preferences.

• Frequency: current recommendation is annual.

• Describe LDCT – Low-Dose CT (CAT) scan:
  • You will need to lie still on a table for about 15 minutes.
  • It is painless.
  • There is radiation, but it is low-dose (equals approximately 15 chest x-rays).
  • Current screening protocol calls for repeating it annually.

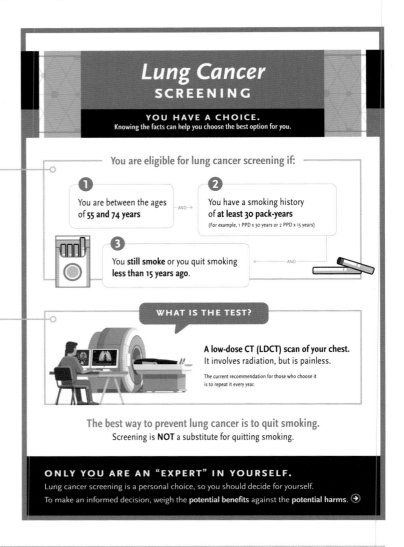

Additional Information

Shared decision making is increasingly being incorporated into standards of care. Medicare requires that patients discuss the benefits and risks of lung cancer screening before proceeding with this[1].

Background[2]

• <u>Lung cancer is the leading cause of cancer death in the US.</u>

• **Annual US Incidence**   Age-adjusted Rates

Male:	111,907	70 per 100,000 population
Female:	100,677	52 per 100,000 population
Total:	212,584	59 per 100,000 population

• **Mortality**   Age-adjusted Rates

Male:	85,658	54 per 100,000 population
Female:	70,518	35 per 100,000 population
Total:	156,176	43 per 100,000 population

• **Age Distribution**
  • Incidence: Ages 40 – 64: 65,462 | 64 per 100,000 persons
    Ages ≥ 65: 146,038 | **329** per 100,000 persons
  • Mortality: Ages 40 – 64: 42,733 | 41 per 100,000 persons
    Ages ≥ 65: 113,032 | **253** per 100,000 persons

Area of Uncertainty

• It is unclear whether engaging in lung cancer screening increases or decreases smoking cessation rates.

Screening benefits

• Lung cancer mortality reduction: 3 per 1000 per 6.5 years

Burdens associated with testing

• **Inconvenience:** Annual testing

• **Cost:** Approximately $250 per scan; usually covered by insurance if patient meets eligibility criteria

Screening Harms

• False Positives per 1000:
  • 365 get additional imaging
  • 25 get a biopsy
  • 3 experience a complication from their biopsy

• Overdiagnosis: 4 per 1000

• Radiation-Induced Conditions: for every 2500 people having three annual LDCTs, there will be 1 death from a cancer <u>caused</u> by the radiation exposure

This chapter is primarily based on data from the National Lung Screening Trial (NLST), a study[3] that was performed at 33 academic centers with highly-trained radiologists and multi-disciplinary teams. Selection criteria and clinical protocols were strictly followed. Failure to follow these in actual clinical practice may yield significantly different outcomes.

Screening outcomes in practice may also be inferior to NLST results because, compared to all eligible patients, NLST participants were on average younger, better educated, and less likely to be current smokers.

1. https://www.medicare.gov/coverage/lung-cancer-screening.html, accessed August 2017

2. Surveillance for Cancer Incidence and Mortality – United States 2013. *MMWR January 27, 2017. Vol. 66. No.4: 1-35.*

3. National Lung Screening Trial Research Team. Reduced Lung-Cancer Mortality with Low-Dose Computed Tomographic Screening. *N Engl J Med 2011;365:395-409.*

Lung Cancer
SCREENING

YOU HAVE A CHOICE.
Knowing the facts can help you choose the best option for you.

You are eligible for lung cancer screening if:

1 You are between the ages of **55 and 74 years**

—AND→

2 You have a smoking history of **at least 30 pack-years**

(For example, 1 PPD x 30 years or 2 PPD x 15 years)

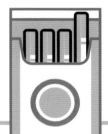

3 You **still smoke** or you quit smoking **less than 15 years ago**.

←AND—

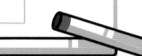

WHAT IS THE TEST?

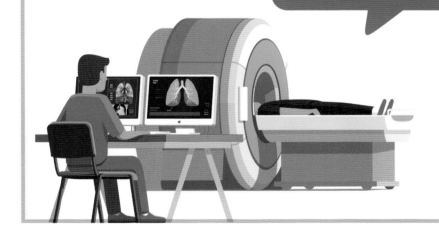

A low-dose CT (LDCT) scan of your chest.
It involves radiation, but is painless.

The current recommendation for those who choose it is to repeat it every year.

The best way to prevent lung cancer is to quit smoking.
Screening is **NOT** a substitute for quitting smoking.

ONLY <u>YOU</u> ARE AN "EXPERT" IN YOURSELF.

Lung cancer screening is a personal choice, so you should decide for yourself.

To make an informed decision, weigh the **potential benefits** against the **potential harms**.

Set the Stage

Share:

★ The column on the left shows what happens (over the next 6.5 years) to 1000 people who choose annual LDCT screening

★ The column on the right shows what happens to 1000 people who do not choose screening.

★ Each dot represents 1 person.

★ You have an **equal chance of being any one** of these 1000 dots.

★ In each group of 1000 people, 960 people will not have or get lung cancer, and 40 (36 + 4) will have or get lung cancer.

★ **4 of the 40 lung cancers are turtle-type cancers:** they will not be diagnosed in the No Screening group —and they will never cause any symptoms or harm for those 4 people.

Explain the meaning of the different color dots.

• Gray: No cancer
• Green: cancer with good outcome
• Black: Cancer that causes death
• Red: Overdiagnosed Cancer (never would have caused any harm if not diagnosed)
• Yellow: False Positive (= no cancer, but abnormal test result)

Review the ANNUAL LDCT SCREENING Section

Share:

• Among the 960 people in the screening group without lung cancer, the **595 gray dots** (62%) represent people who will have normal CTs, and they will be reassured by this, but ...

★ The 365 yellow dots (38%) represent people without lung cancer who will have false positive CTs.

★ **Explain the false positives**: things that are seen on the CT that raise a concern of a problem, but after further testing we learn that it was really nothing.

  • All 365 of these people get extra testing; for most of them it is just additional CT scans, but:

    • **25 will have a biopsy** (a surgical procedure to remove a sample of the lung to examine it under a microscope).

    • Among these 25, **3 people will have a complication from the biopsy**, often requiring them to receive treatments in the hospital.

• Among the 36 people with bad cancers (bears and grenades), the 18 green dots represent people who will **survive** and the **18 black dots** represent people who will **die** of lung cancer. This is the prime benefit of screening, because 3 fewer die compared to the No Screening group.

★ **The 4 red dots represent cases of** overdiagnosed lung cancers: turtle-type cancers that were found only because of the screening.

  • Because these never would have caused symptoms or harm, there is no possible benefit from diagnosing or treating them. Cancer treatments always cause harms. These people will die from something other than lung cancer, though they will suffer from the diagnosis and treatment of lung cancer.

★ **REMEMBER:** At the time of choosing screening, you have an equal chance of being any of these 1000 dots.

Review the NO LDCT SCREENING Section

Share:

★ The 960 gray dots represent people who do not have or get lung cancer. They have no testing and no problems.

• There are 36 people who will have or get a bad lung cancer (bear- and grenade-type). After developing symptoms, they will get diagnosed with and treated for lung cancer.

  ★ the 15 green dots represent people who will survive and the 21 black dots represent people who will **die** of lung cancer, **3 more than in the screened group.**

★ **The 4 green dots in their own section represent turtle-type cancers**, which will never cause any symptoms or harm. Because there is no screening in this group, they will never be found, so these 4 people will not be harmed by unnecessary treatments.

Did you know?

Tobacco smoking causes 90% of lung cancers in men and 78% of lung cancers in women.

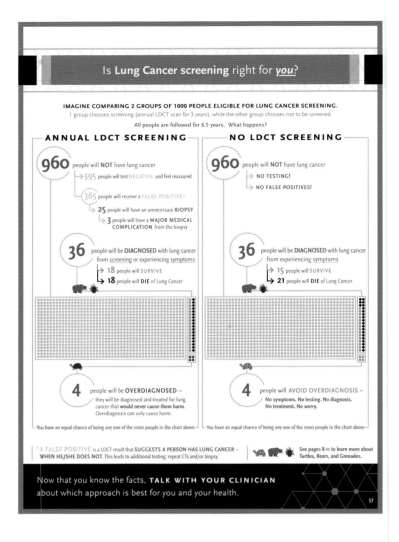

Summary

No screening:

⊗ 3 extra people die of lung cancer
⊘ Everyone avoids unnecessary testing
⊘ 4 people avoid unnecessary treatment for lung cancer

Screening:

⊘ 3 fewer people die of lung cancer
⊗ 4 people diagnosed with and treated unnecessarily for turtle-type, harmless lung cancers
⊗ 365 people have false positive tests
⊗ 25 have a biopsy
⊗ 3 have a complication

Debrief

State:

• "We reviewed a lot of information today."

Ask:

• "Are there are any parts of it you would like to go over again?"
★ "Do you have any questions?"
★ "Do you feel ready to make a decision?"
• "Would you like to talk about quitting smoking?" (if appropriate)

Is **Lung Cancer screening** right for *you?*

IMAGINE COMPARING 2 GROUPS OF 1000 PEOPLE ELIGIBLE FOR LUNG CANCER SCREENING.

1 group chooses screening (annual LDCT scan for 3 years), while the other group chooses not to be screened.

All people are followed for 6.5 years. What happens?

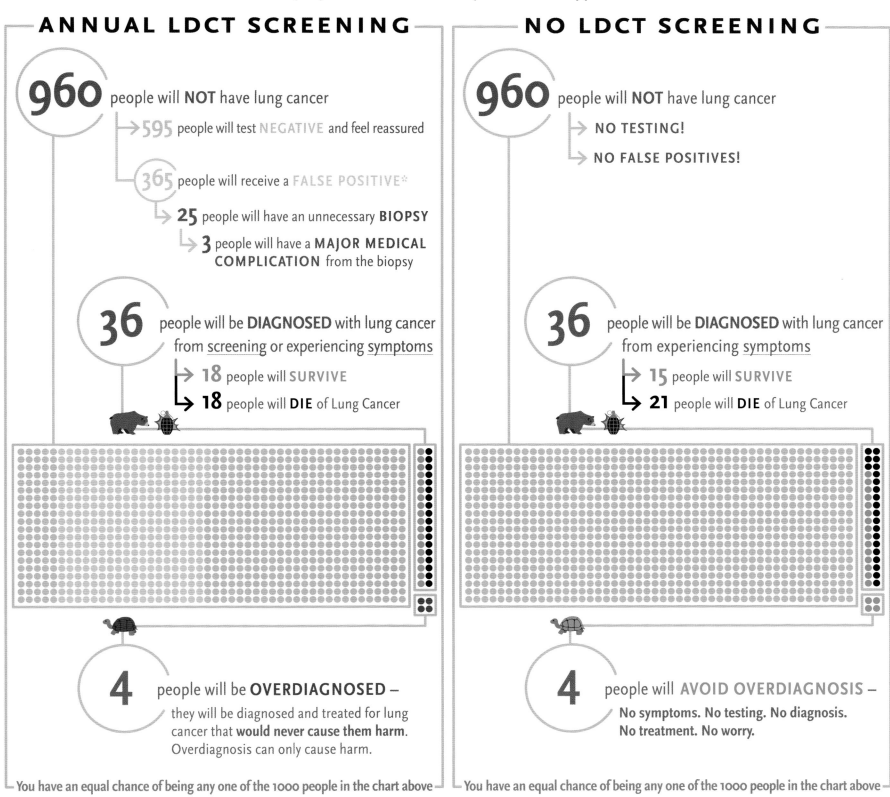

ANNUAL LDCT SCREENING

960 people will **NOT** have lung cancer

→ **595** people will test NEGATIVE and feel reassured

365 people will receive a FALSE POSITIVE*

↳ **25** people will have an unnecessary **BIOPSY**

↳ **3** people will have a **MAJOR MEDICAL COMPLICATION** from the biopsy

36 people will be **DIAGNOSED** with lung cancer from screening or experiencing symptoms

→ **18** people will SURVIVE
→ **18** people will **DIE** of Lung Cancer

4 people will be **OVERDIAGNOSED** –
they will be diagnosed and treated for lung cancer that **would never cause them harm**. Overdiagnosis can only cause harm.

You have an equal chance of being any one of the 1000 people in the chart above

NO LDCT SCREENING

960 people will **NOT** have lung cancer

→ NO TESTING!

→ NO FALSE POSITIVES!

36 people will be **DIAGNOSED** with lung cancer from experiencing symptoms

→ **15** people will SURVIVE
→ **21** people will **DIE** of Lung Cancer

4 people will AVOID OVERDIAGNOSIS –
No symptoms. No testing. No diagnosis. No treatment. No worry.

You have an equal chance of being any one of the 1000 people in the chart above

---

*A FALSE POSITIVE is a LDCT result that **SUGGESTS A PERSON HAS LUNG CANCER –
WHEN HE/SHE DOES NOT.** This leads to additional testing: repeat CTs and/or biopsy.

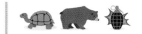 See pages 8-11 to learn more about
Turtles, Bears, and Grenades.

Now that you know the facts, **TALK WITH YOUR CLINICIAN**
about which approach is best for you and your health.

Prostate Cancer Screening

Clinician Talking Points & Discussion Guide

Below, please find suggested questions and talking points to help guide your conversation with your patient.
If a bullet has a ★ next to it, we <u>highly recommend</u> including this in your discussion.

Introduction

Ask:

★ "Is this a good time for you to discuss prostate cancer screening?"

• "Is there anyone else you would like to participate in the conversation, such as a family member?"

Review KNOW THE FACTS

Share:

❶ 14% of men will get prostate cancer at some point.

★ Prostate cancer is more common as men get older:

  • Median age at diagnosis: 66. Median age at death: 80.[3]
  • Among men age 50 years, 2.1 % will be diagnosed with prostate cancer in the next 10 years.[4]
  • Among men age 60 years, 5.8 % will be diagnosed with prostate cancer in the next 10 years.[4]
  • Among men age 70 years, 6.9 % will be diagnosed with prostate cancer in the next 10 years.[4]

❷ Many cases never cause harm. You may wish to explain about turtle-type cancers here.
See pages 8-11.

❸ A blood test, called PSA, is available.

• Because of the balance of harms to benefits, many men decide <u>not</u> to have a PSA screening test.

Review EXPERTS RECOMMEND

Share:

• There is now greater agreement among guideline recommendations for prostate cancer screening with PSA than ever before.

★ All the recommendations place a high priority on:
  • Informing men of the benefits and harms
  • Facilitating decision making based on individual patient values and preferences

★ Evidence suggests that longer screening intervals preserve most of the benefits of screening, while reducing many of the harms

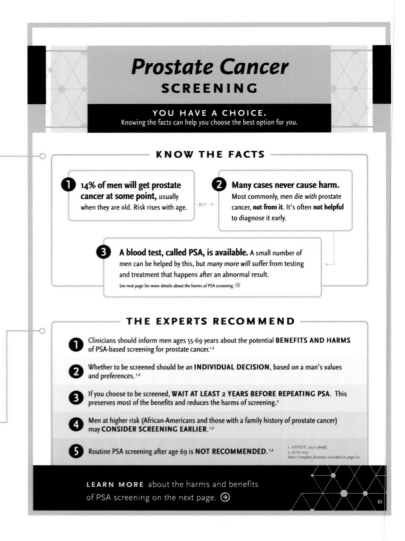

You may wish to share this table, which shows substantial variation by race:

• US Prostate Cancer Rates **per 100,000 Men** per Year (2014)[5]

RACE	INCIDENCE	MORTALITY
African-American	154	38
White	87	18
Hispanic	80	15
Asian	46	8
TOTAL	**96**	**19**

Summary

Share:

• Many prostate cancers are indolent (Turtles)

• There is no all-cause mortality benefit from PSA screening.

• The prostate cancer mortality benefit of screening is small.

• Many men decide against PSA screening due to the high rates of:
  • False Positives
  • Overdiagnosed Cancers

1. USPSTF 2017 Draft Recommendation Statement. Accessed August 20, 2017 at https://www.uspreventiveservicestaskforce.org/Page/Document/draft-recommendation-statement/prostate-cancer-screening1

2. American Urological Association. 2015. Accessed August 8, 2017. http://www.auanet.org/guidelines/early-detection-of-prostate-cancer-(2013-reviewed-and-validity-confirmed-2015)

3. SEER 2010-2014. https://seer.cancer.gov/statfacts/html/prost.html Accessed July 15, 2017.

4. Accessed at https://www.cdc.gov/cancer/prostate/statistics/age.htm where the following sources were cited: Howlader N, Noone AM, Krapcho M, Garshell J, Miller D, Altekruse SF, Kosary CL, Yu M, Ruhl J, Tatalovich Z, Mariotto A, Lewis DR, Chen HS, Feuer EJ, Cronin KA (eds). SEER Cancer Statistics Review, 1975–2012, National Cancer Institute. Bethesda, MD, http://seer.cancer.gov/csr/1975_2012/browse_csr.php?sectionSEL=23&pageSEL=sect_23_table.10.html, based on November 2014 SEER data submission, posted to the SEER Web site, April 2015.

5. U.S. Cancer Statistics Working Group. United States Cancer Statistics: 1999-2014 Incidence and Mortality Web-based Report. Atlanta: U.S. Department of Health and Human Services, Centers for Disease Control and Prevention and National Cancer Institute; 2017. Available at: www.cdc.gov/uscs.

Prostate Cancer
SCREENING

KNOW THE FACTS

1 **14% of men will get prostate cancer at some point,** usually when they are old. Risk rises with age.

—BUT→

2 **Many cases never cause harm.** Most commonly, men die *with* prostate cancer, **not from it.** It's often **not helpful** to diagnose it early.

3 **A blood test, called PSA, is available.** A small number of men can be helped by this, but *many more will suffer* from testing and treatment that happens after an abnormal result.

See next page for more details about the harms of PSA screening. ⊘

THE EXPERTS RECOMMEND

1 Clinicians should inform men ages 55-69 years about the potential **BENEFITS AND HARMS** of PSA-based screening for prostate cancer.[1,2]

2 Whether to be screened should be an **INDIVIDUAL DECISION**, based on a man's values and preferences. [1,2]

3 If you choose to be screened, **WAIT AT LEAST 2 YEARS BEFORE REPEATING PSA.** This preserves most of the benefits and reduces the harms of screening.[2]

4 Men at higher risk (African-Americans and those with a family history of prostate cancer) may **CONSIDER SCREENING EARLIER.** [1,2]

5 Routine PSA screening after age 69 is **NOT RECOMMENDED.** [1,2]

1. USPSTF, 2017 (draft)
2. AUA 2015
Note: Complete footnotes included on page 60

LEARN MORE about the harms and benefits of PSA screening on the next page. ➡

Set the Stage

Share:

- Each chart shows 1000 men and what happens to them over 11 years based on whether they choose regular PSA screening or not.

★ In each group, there are 890 men without prostate cancer and 110 men with prostate cancer: 66 with potentially bad cancers (Bears and Grenades) and 44 indolent (Turtle) cancers.

★ The 44 Turtle cancers in the No Screening group are never diagnosed — and they never cause any symptoms or problems.

Explain the meaning of the different color dots. (About 5% of men have some form of color blindness, so you may want to inquire about that.)

- Gray: No cancer
- Green: cancer with good outcome
- Black: Cancer that causes death
- Red: Overdiagnosed Cancer (never would have caused any harm if not diagnosed)
- Yellow: False Positive (= no cancer, but abnormal test result)

Review the REGULAR PSA SCREENING Section

Share:

- These are men who get regular (e.g., every 1 or 2 years) PSA testing.

- Among the 890 men without prostate cancer, the 780 gray dots represent men who will have normal PSA tests, and they will be reassured by this, but ...

★ The 110 yellow dots represent men who experience false positives: even though they do not have prostate cancer, their PSA test will be abnormal.

  - 100 of these men will go on to have a biopsy, and 32 of them will have a significant problem from the biopsy, such as infection, bleeding or problems urinating.

- Because of symptoms or PSA testing, 66 men will be diagnosed with prostate cancer – in most cases earlier than in the No Screening group.

  - After treatment, the 62 green dots represent men who will survive, and the 4 black dots represent men who will die of prostate cancer, so 1 man in this group of 1000 avoids dying of prostate cancer because of PSA testing.

★ The 44 red dots represent cases of overdiagnosed prostate cancer: men with indolent, turtle-type cancers who get diagnosed with and treated for prostate cancer because of their PSA screening.

  ★ Treatment for prostate cancer often causes incontinence and impotence.

Emphasize:

★ Your patient has an equal chance of being any one of the 1000 men represented in either chart.

Review the NO PSA SCREENING Section

Share:

★ There is no routine testing in this group.

★ Because of symptoms, 66 men will be diagnosed with prostate cancer.

  - After treatment, the 61 green dots represent men who will survive, and the 5 black dots represent men who will die of prostate cancer, 1 more than in the screened group

★ The 44 green dots in their own section represent men with indolent, turtle-type cancers. They will never learn they cancer, and their cancers will never cause them any problem.

Emphasize:

★ Your patient has an equal chance of being any one of the 1000 men represented in either chart.

Although 1 man per 1000 may avoid dying *from prostate cancer* due to PSA screening, there is **no all-cause mortality benefit**.

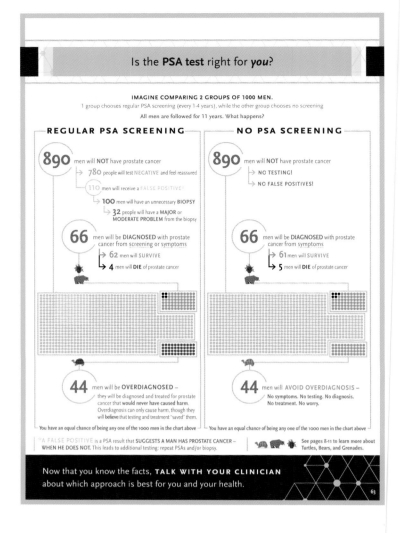

Summary

No screening:

- ⊗ 1 extra man dies of prostate cancer
- ⊘ Everyone avoids unnecessary testing
- ⊘ 44 men avoid unnecessary diagnosis and treatment for turtle-type, harmless prostate cancers

Screening:

- ⊘ 1 extra man avoids dying from prostate cancer
- ⊗ 44 men get diagnosed and treated unnecessarily for turtle-type, harmless prostate cancers
- ⊗ 110 men have false positive test results
- ⊗ 100 men have a prostate biopsy
- ⊗ 32 men have a complication from the biopsy

Debrief

State:

- "We reviewed a lot of information today."

Ask:

- "Are there are any parts you would like me to go over again?"

★ "Do you have any questions?"

★ "Before you make a decision, you might want to consider questions such as:

  - Do I want to know if I have prostate cancer?
  - Would I want to have a biopsy if my PSA test were abnormal?
  - How would I feel if I learned it was a false positive?
  - Knowing that prostate cancer treatments often cause incontinence and impotence, how willing am I to accept the risk of overdiagnosis?
  - How would I feel if I didn't choose screening and later learned that I had prostate cancer?"

- "Do you feel ready to make a decision about PSA screening?"

The numbers in the chart are adapted from ERSPC, the European Randomized Study of Screening for Prostate Cancer, which included 182,000 men.

Schroder FH, Hugosson J, Roobol MJ, et al. Prostate-cancer mortality at 11 years of follow-up. *N Engl J Med* 2012;366:981-90.

Is the **PSA test** right for *you*?

IMAGINE COMPARING 2 GROUPS OF 1000 MEN.

1 group chooses regular PSA screening (every 1-4 years), while the other group chooses no screening

All men are followed for 11 years. What happens?

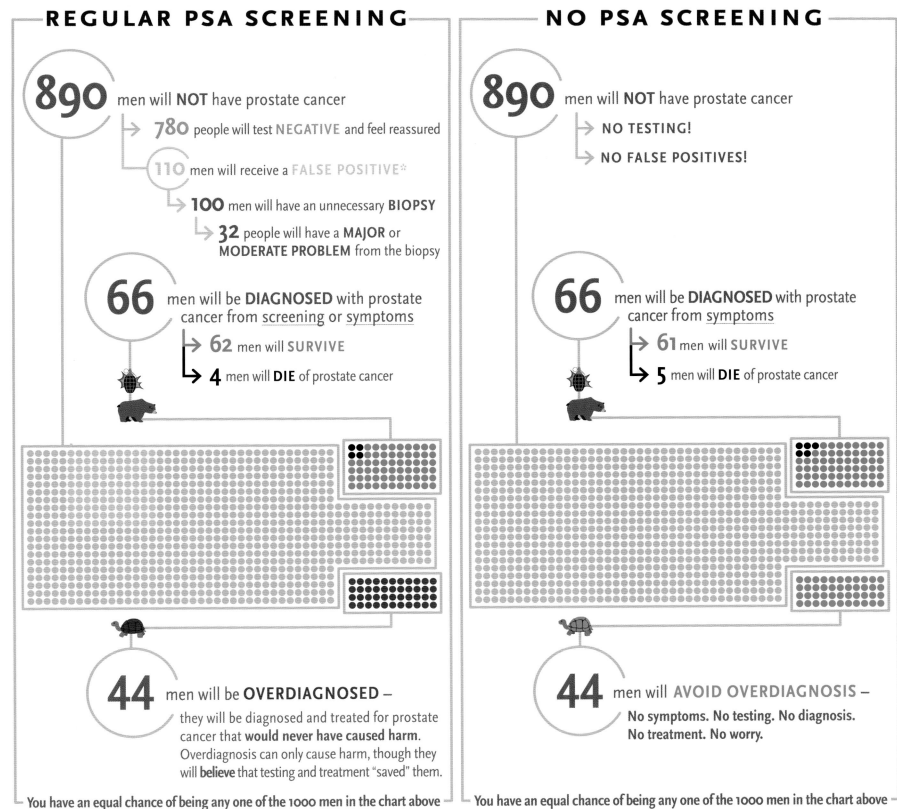

REGULAR PSA SCREENING

890 men will **NOT** have prostate cancer
→ **780** people will test NEGATIVE and feel reassured
→ **110** men will receive a FALSE POSITIVE*
→ **100** men will have an unnecessary **BIOPSY**
→ **32** people will have a **MAJOR** or **MODERATE PROBLEM** from the biopsy

66 men will be **DIAGNOSED** with prostate cancer from <u>screening</u> or <u>symptoms</u>
→ **62** men will SURVIVE
→ **4** men will **DIE** of prostate cancer

44 men will be **OVERDIAGNOSED** –
they will be diagnosed and treated for prostate cancer that **would never have caused harm**. Overdiagnosis can only cause harm, though they will **believe** that testing and treatment "saved" them.

You have an equal chance of being any one of the 1000 men in the chart above

NO PSA SCREENING

890 men will **NOT** have prostate cancer
→ **NO TESTING!**
→ **NO FALSE POSITIVES!**

66 men will be **DIAGNOSED** with prostate cancer from <u>symptoms</u>
→ **61** men will SURVIVE
→ **5** men will **DIE** of prostate cancer

44 men will AVOID OVERDIAGNOSIS –
No symptoms. No testing. No diagnosis. No treatment. No worry.

You have an equal chance of being any one of the 1000 men in the chart above

*A FALSE POSITIVE is a PSA result that **SUGGESTS A MAN HAS PROSTATE CANCER – WHEN HE DOES NOT.** This leads to additional testing: repeat PSAs and/or biopsy.

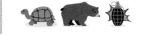 **See pages 8-11 to learn more about Turtles, Bears, and Grenades.**

Now that you know the facts, **TALK WITH YOUR CLINICIAN** about which approach is best for you and your health.